KU-605-352

keto-
green ™

Includes more
than 50
delicious recipes!

16

DR ANNA CABECA

Quercus

Published in the US in 2020 by Ballantine Books, an imprint of Random House,
a division of Penguin Random House LLC, New York.

First published in Great Britain by

Quercus Editions Ltd
Carmelite House
50 Victoria Embankment
London EC4Y 0DZ

An Hachette UK company

Copyright © Anna Cabeca 2020

The moral right of Anna Cabeca to be
identified as the author of this work has been
asserted in accordance with the
Copyright, Designs and Patents Act, 1988.

All rights reserved. No part of this publication
may be reproduced or transmitted in any form
or by any means, electronic or mechanical,
including photocopy, recording, or any
information storage and retrieval system,
without permission in writing from the publisher.

A CIP catalogue record for this book is available
from the British Library.

TPB ISBN 978 1 52941 059 4
Ebook ISBN 978 1 52941 060 0

Every effort has been made to contact copyright holders.
However, the publishers will be glad to rectify in future editions
any inadvertent omissions brought to their attention.

Quercus Editions Ltd hereby exclude all liability to the extent
permitted by law for any errors or omissions in this book and
for any loss, damage or expense (whether direct or indirect) suffered
by a third party relying on any information contained in this book.

If you have a medical condition or suspect one, consult your GP before following
Keto-Green 16. Nothing in this book is intended to replace or override any medical advice
or treatment you may be receiving. Author and publisher accept no responsibility for
health outcomes from the methods in this book.

Book design by Diane Hobbing

10 9 8 7 6 5 4 3 2 1

Printed and bound in Great Britain by Clays Ltd, Elcograf S.p.A.

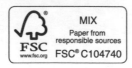

Papers used by Quercus Editions Ltd are from well-managed forests and other responsible sources.

South Dublin Libraries

www.southdublinlibraries.ie

2 0 OCT 2020

KETO-GREEN 16

Also by Dr Anna Cabeca

The Hormone Fix

To my loving daughters, Brittany, Amanda, Amira, and Avamarie. You inspire me to live healthier every day and share these lessons with faith and love.

FOREWORD

David Perlmutter, MD

According to the National Center for Health Statistics, American life expectancy started to decline in 2014—for the first time in American history. This despite the fact that the United States has the highest spending per capita on healthcare in the world.

What's cutting our lives short? Both here in America and in locales around the world where life expectancy is also dipping, the culprit isn't accidents or even infectious disease.

What is killing humans across the globe are chronic degenerative conditions like diabetes, cancer, coronary artery disease, and Alzheimer's. Though this might at first seem like a list of different and unrelated diseases, they do all share a common denominator, a root cause: systemic inflammation.

And what contributes significantly to inflammation? Our Western diet.

A Western diet is generally one that is high in ultraprocessed foods, sugar, and refined carbohydrates, while low in dietary fiber and healthful fat.

As such, we are witnessing a worldwide spread of a dietary trend that *augments* inflammation. Add to this the fact that it has now been scientifically established that inflammation effectively reduces our access to the prefrontal cortex. This means more-impulsive thinking and poor decision-making. Indeed, correlation with higher markers of inflammation is seen not only in diabetes, hypertension, and renal failure but also in "diseases of despair" like depression, alcoholism, and obesity.

Our most valuable tool in combating chronic inflammation is making good choices about the foods we consume.

And clearly, there now exists robust science that is strongly supportive of a ketogenic diet for accomplishing this goal.

A diet that will promote ketosis is a diet that not only helps lower inflammation but, more specifically, also helps in the reduction of excess body fat, enhances energy production, and helps reestablish insulin sensitivity, thereby helping to reduce risk for type II diabetes.

Because of these and other benefits, public interest in "going keto" has grown exponentially.

But despite the seeming simplicity of ketogenic eating—cutting carbs and increasing dietary fat—many people have a hard time with commonly experienced side effects. Because of the mantra to "cut out all carbs," many people get constipated. Due to mineral deficiencies of the classic ketogenic diet (most often potassium and magnesium), some people experience "keto flu."

In the pages that follow, however, Dr. Anna Cabeca presents a highly researched and nuanced approach to a ketogenic diet that significantly increases the likelihood of getting into ketosis while decreasing the likelihood of these and other unwanted side effects. Her plan provides you the fiber you'll need to stave off constipation, as well as mineral-rich vegetables that will surely add to both the efficacy and tolerability of her program.

Our goal with respect to nutrition is to consume the highest-quality nutrient-dense foods available while targeting inflammation.

Keto-Green 16 is a powerful program for accomplishing these goals and paving the way for lasting health, longevity, and disease resistance.

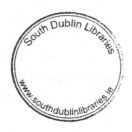
South Dublin Libraries
www.southdublinlibraries.ie

CONTENTS

INTRODUCTION

Welcome to Keto-Green 16! The next sixteen days are going to be exciting, encouraging, and uplifting as you begin to drop pounds—perhaps up to a pound a day!—and lose inches around your waist, without cravings or hunger. At the same time, you'll begin to feel mentally and physically energized like never before. And, I predict, you will feel a dramatic improvement in your digestive health, your sleep, and, even more excitingly, your mood.

All of these things happen when you go Keto-Green—a scientifically validated, breakthrough way of eating that combines a fat-melting ketogenic diet (low in carbs, high in good fats, moderate in protein) with health-boosting alkaline-rich foods. You'll also incorporate intermittent fasting into your routine, going without food for roughly sixteen hours (mostly overnight). It's the healthiest way to fast, and its impact on fat-burning and metabolism is remarkable.

I understand that you might be a little skeptical about considering yet another diet. You've probably removed unhealthy foods from your diet before. You've exercised as much as you can. You've yo-yo dieted, sometimes gaining back more than you originally lost. And then there's the dreaded, hard-to-lose belly fat. Through it all, you're still unable to shed as many pounds as you want, and you can't see the results of your efforts and hard work. And if you do see results, they seem to be only temporary.

What's the problem? What's going wrong with your body? Why is it so hard to lose weight—especially as you get older and, for many women, enter menopause?

I get it. Do I ever! At age thirty-eight, I weighed more than 240 pounds, with a lot of it abdominal fat. Then I lost one of my children, my toddler, Garrett, and wasn't in any mental or emotional shape to focus on losing weight. But after taking a healing journey around the world in the wake of that tragedy, I eventually got below 150 pounds, got pregnant again (after being declared infertile), and was able to stay at that healthy weight for ten years.

Then, when I was forty-eight, menopause hit, and I quickly gained twenty pounds, seemingly overnight. It was a time in my life of toxic romantic relationships (like the time I got engaged to the wrong guy), brain fog, near-bankruptcy, and more. The stress, combined with my changing hormones, made it seemingly impossible to get thin and feel well.

The more I talked to my patients and saw how their stories mirrored mine, I realized I wasn't alone—and neither are you! I was in a metabolic stall and mental fog brought on by hormones. I had to understand what was happening in this peri-menopausal time period to my body and my mind.

I was determined to figure out why it's so hard to get lasting results and how to conquer this stubborn problem—and do it quickly.

Brain, Body, and Belly

It turns out that the missing link in getting to and staying at a healthy weight is your brain. Your brain has significant power over your hormones, and these affect your weight, your metabolism, and your appetite. If there is a disconnect between your brain and your body, your hormones will not function optimally—a condition I call neuroendocrine vulnerability—and it will be challenging to lose weight and keep it off. But we can get to our happy weight, and we can do it effortlessly. So hang in there with me.

Hormones are chemicals that conduct an intricate symphony of messaging throughout our bodies, regulating everything from sleep to sex, mood to energy, mobility to growth.

Several hormones play a huge role in hunger and its opposite: satiety, the happy feeling of being full and satisfied after a meal. Others help the body burn fat and reduce weight, even belly fat. You may already be familiar with insulin, a hormone that tells your muscle cells to take in glucose (blood sugar) from the bloodstream.

Our reproductive hormones are involved in weight too. As we age, our bodies slowly decrease the production of estrogen, progesterone, DHEA, and testosterone, causing more fat tissue to form around our middle.

Even stress hormones like cortisol get into the act. Because most of us are constantly under stress, cortisol stays spiked in the body. Excess cortisol triggers the release of energy in the form of fat and glucose. Ultimately, the fat is redeposited as pudge around the belly, near the liver, forming an unhealthy type of fat called visceral fat.

Most people haven't heard of the hormone adiponectin, which controls glucose levels and fat burning.

What all hormones have in common is that they are in contact with the brain. By making us feel more or less hungry, speeding up or slowing down our metabolism, or controlling the burning of fat, these hormones, when in balance, interact with the brain to make tiny course corrections to help keep our weight within a healthy range.

Once you get balanced and your hormones are working in sync with your brain, you'll resolve neuroendocrine vulnerability. As a result, you'll more easily burn fat, develop toned muscles, and stay in fat-burning mode even when you're not moving.

So the key is to train your brain and balance your hormones to work for and with your body, instead of against it—and get sexy and slim in the process.

And with my Keto-Green diet, you can do it in just sixteen days. Isn't that great news?

What to Expect

On Keto-Green 16, you'll experience and discover how to:

- **Lose weight rapidly.** This diet promotes ketosis, a process in which your body starts burning stored fat, and does so quickly. It also keeps your blood sugar steady all day so that you avoid hunger and cravings. It's a great kick-start to move you off a plateau, gain willpower, and get results fast. In two studies I conducted at North Florida Integrative Medicine in Gainesville, Florida, in 2019, with forty-three people, the participants lost anywhere from half a pound to nearly one pound a day—without feeling hungry or fatigued. What's more, they felt better and had reduced symptom scores overall!

- **Strip off those last five or ten pounds.** Here's where dieters really struggle—those final stubborn pounds that block you from getting to your happy weight. It's a common problem you've probably encountered in your quest for lower numbers on the scale and a shapelier image in the mirror. But don't worry. I've had many clients who wanted to get rid of those obstinate five or ten pounds, and they did it within sixteen days.

- **Get a tinier waist.** No one likes having a flabby belly, yet tummy fat and muffin tops can often be the hardest places on the body to pry loose the pudge. Belly fat not only is unsightly, but also can be deadly as we get older because it contributes to a higher risk of heart disease, diabetes, and chronic illness, more so than any other fat in your body. Keto-Green 16 helps you lose weight specifically from the abdominal area and keep it off for good, because it targets poorly balanced hormones that pile pounds on your waistline. In my studies, participants lost an average of 2.25 inches around their midsections in only sixteen days. How's that for waist reduction?

- **Flush out toxins.** Every day we're exposed to toxins and unnatural substances in our environment—toxins the body likes to store in fat tissue, other tissues, and various organs, affecting their operation. Many of these toxins are hormone-disrupting chemicals that influence how much weight we gain or lose. They have been found to create more and bigger fat cells, or trick the brain into making us eat more.

  Fortunately, our bodies are good housekeepers, automatically doing the job of cleaning out or neutralizing toxins through the colon, liver, kidneys, lungs, lymph system, and skin. But the body needs help to do its cleanup job. This plan provides naturally detoxifying foods and alkaline foods, along with intermittent fasting, to rid the body of these unnatural chemicals so we can lose weight for good.

- **Exercise less but get more results.** With my sixteen-minute workout, you'll learn how to perform high-intensity interval training (HIIT), a type of workout that uses short bursts of strenuous activity to ramp up your heart rate and boost your fitness. Interval training is the perfect companion to the Keto-Green 16 diet because this type of workout also regulates several hunger and weight-gain hormones.

- **Enjoy greater physical energy.** On Keto-Green 16 your body starts burning more fat for energy, rather than carbs or sugar. This occurs because without carby or sugary foods, your body taps into fat stores for fuel. And by avoiding sugary foods, which cause fleeting energy highs followed by fast crashes, you won't have those energy slumps that lead to a lack of productivity and concentration.

- **Develop sharper thinking.** Your brain is a hungry organ, constantly taking energy from the bloodstream in order to send and receive electrical signals twenty-four hours a day, creating complex thoughts and emotions.

  The brain possesses the ability to metabolize glucose and ketones for energy. The best source of glucose is from a diet rich in low-carb vegetables and fruit—like the Keto-Green 16 diet. The brain, however, hates glucose obtained from refined sugar. This kind of sugar is known to ruin cognitive function and memory. You won't be eating any brain-destructive sugar on this plan!

On the Keto-Green 16 diet, you'll be limiting your carbs to 40 grams daily or less. Consequently, your hungry brain dials 911 and says, "Hey, I need more glucose fast!" Your liver answers the call by converting stored fatty acids into ketone bodies to serve as a backup fuel source. They are shuttled to the brain to keep it happy, satisfied, and operating at maximum capacity.

Compared to glucose, ketone bodies are an ideal energy source for the brain. They supply more energy per unit of oxygen consumed by the brain, provide that energy at a faster rate, help regulate weight-control hormones like leptin and insulin, and reduce free radicals associated with brain inflammation. The net effect of ketone bodies on the brain is sharper thinking and prevention of neurological disorders and conditions.

The brain loves to run on these natural chemicals! Across the board, nearly everyone in my studies reported sharper mental focus, clearer thinking, and vanishing brain fog. This shift in fuel source from glucose to ketones is especially essential if you're in perimenopause or postmenopause.

- **Monitor how well your body is reacting to the diet.** By using interpretive tools such as test strips to measure ketosis and alkalinity, a monitoring system for glucose that does not require pricking your finger, and your scale (which will no longer be the enemy), you'll have quick and reliable feedback on how your body is functioning and adapting to my plan.

- **Create tasty, filling menus.** Using my delicious Keto-Green 16 recipes, made from ingredients available at your grocery store (no obscure specialty foods), you'll love every bite as you watch the pounds fall off.

Keto-Green 16 is a take-the-bull-by-the-horns approach to weight loss. It doesn't come with a guarantee of no effort on your part. It calls for a commitment to eating specific fat-burning and alkaline-boosting foods, intermittent fasting, and getting more active. Yes, I'd say it's challenging, but what doesn't challenge you won't change you! Indeed, what's challenging is always worth doing—especially for looking great, feeling energetic, and enjoying life more. Start with an open mind and let the rapid changes Keto-Green 16 produces in the way you look and the way you feel be the indicators of whether it is worth that effort.

I know you've had frustrations with diets throughout your life. So have I. But no more. The benefits of this plan are so great that you'll embrace it as a way of life.

Let's get going. You can do this!

—Anna Cabeca, DO

Part One

Fix the Hormones That Control
Your Brain, Body, and Belly

Chapter 1

So . . . You Can't Lose Weight?

In my work as a physician and hormone expert, I hear from women (and men too) all the time that no matter what they do, the pounds won't go. They see their midsection thickening, even if they're eating healthfully and exercising. They've had to buy bigger clothes to compensate for weight landing on their tummies and hips. As successful as they are in other areas of their lives, they feel defeated when it comes to weight loss. And they beat themselves up over it.

Right now, normal-weight Americans constitute a minority. Two out of three adults and one out of three children are either overweight or obese. This crisis has reached epidemic proportions in adults, and it's about to do the same in kids.

A big problem behind this epidemic is that for too long, overweight people were told: "Just eat less, have smaller meals and more frequent meals, have better willpower, and you'll be fine." But today we know that these recommendations greatly oversimplify the issue.

I know that your creeping weight gain is not because you're plowing through bags of candy. It is because your hormones are shifting and have become unbalanced. They are working against you and your metabolism, and against your sincerest efforts to lose weight. So it's not your fault if you have trouble shedding pounds. Stop blaming yourself. It's your hormones.

Two Kinds of Fat

As we get older, part of the weight we put on, especially during menopause, is stored as subcutaneous fat—fat that's just under the skin in our thighs, hips, tummy, and elsewhere. And some will be packed away as visceral fat—near our vital organs in the abdominal area, as well as around our blood vessels.

Subcutaneous fat and visceral fat differ not only in their bodily position but also in the threat they pose to your well-being. Laboratory analyses of visceral fat cells have revealed that they're more biologically active than subcutaneous fat cells. Fatty acids and triglycerides (blood fats) move quickly into visceral fat cells, which serve as short-term storehouses for fats. If you're eating excess calories, some of them will be readily deposited in visceral fat, and your waistline will thicken—possibly to a dangerous width.

What constitutes "dangerous"? For your best health, your waist should be less than 35 inches around for women, and less than 40 inches for men. If it's larger than that, you may want to talk with your doctor, because higher waist circumference is associated with a greater risk of problems such as heart disease, high blood pressure, and diabetes.

This weight gain can creep up even while you're maintaining the same diet and exercise routine, and it's very frustrating. It's enough to make you want to throw in the towel, stop trying to get trim, and accept the stubborn weight as inevitable.

But it's not inevitable.

Fluctuating Hormones

If you are among the many women who have tried different diets and exercised diligently but have not lost weight, you probably have a hormonal imbalance. When certain hormone levels change or drop—as they do in the years leading up to menopause—they encourage the body to store fat.

To resolve this problem and get in shape, you must address these hormonal imbalances. Any diet you try to follow that does not tackle hormones will not work, at least not in the long term, and you'll be right back where you started, possibly with more unwanted pounds.

Hormones are chemical messengers, and more than 150 of them run through your body. They impact many functions in your body, including metabolism, reproduction, blood sugar levels, blood pressure, energy levels, kidney function, sleep patterns, aging, appetite, and sex drive.

When it comes to hormones, your brain is command central. The brain prompts the production of hormones via three small but powerful endocrine glands in the brain: the pituitary gland, the hypothalamus, and the pineal gland.

Known as the master gland, the pituitary gland produces hormones that act on the adrenal glands, thyroid gland, ovaries, and testes, which in turn produce other hormones. Through secretion of its hormones, the pituitary gland orchestrates metabolism, growth, sexual maturation, reproduction, blood pressure, and many other vital physical functions and processes.

The hypothalamus is the link between the endocrine and nervous systems. It produces releasing and inhibiting hormones, which stop and start the production of other hormones throughout the body. Some of these hormones include anti-diuretic hormone (ADH), which increases water absorption into the blood by the kidneys; corticotropin-releasing hormone (CRH), which stimulates the adrenals to release cortisol; growth-hormone-releasing hormone (GHRH), which is involved in the production of growth hormone; oxytocin, the bonding hormone; and other hormones involved in the function of the ovaries and testes, breast milk production, and the release of thyroid hormones.

The hypothalamus is in charge of the autonomic nervous system. As the name suggests, this system involves functions that are automatic, not requiring our conscious awareness. Examples of autonomic functions are breathing, hunger, and body temperature.

The pineal gland produces melatonin, a hormone that helps us sleep, age more gracefully, and maintain our circadian rhythm (a clock of sorts, in which our physiological processes are synced to the twenty-four-hour solar cycle of light and dark). Quality sleep and a normal circadian rhythm keep us healthy, and they balance hormones such as cortisol to help us maintain a healthy weight.

These glands and the hormones they produce rarely work solo; instead, they talk to each other and work together. What's more, a dip in the amount of one hormone interferes with other hormones in a domino effect that can throw a host of bodily functions off-kilter. But when in harmony, your hormones function properly, you enjoy good health, your brain is sharp, and your weight is more easily controlled. And you'll have a slimmer, more toned tummy.

The Weight-Control Hormones

To balance your hormones, you need to understand which ones are involved in weight gain and metabolism, why they might be out of whack, and how to correct them. There are thirteen usual suspects:

Estrogen
Progesterone
Testosterone
DHEA
Insulin
Glucagon
Leptin
Ghrelin
Adiponectin
Cortisol
Oxytocin
Thyroid
Growth hormone

Yes, this looks like a long, formidable list. But don't worry: You might have deficiencies in just a few, or several. Everyone is different.

The hormonal changes we experience during our forties and fifties are why so many patients come in complaining about unexpected weight gain and say: "But Dr. Anna, I am not doing anything differently and I'm still gaining weight!" It's your hormones' fault, not yours.

Take Marlene, for example. She was low in only estrogen and progesterone and high in cortisol, according to her hormonal panels. Although she lifted weights regularly and ate healthy foods, she could not lose weight around menopause, and her waist began to gradually thicken. After reviewing her tests, her doctor advised that her number-one priority was diet. Specifically, she had to curb carbohydrates (pasta, breads, even grains). The doctor explained that, hormonally, Marlene's body simply could no longer burn carbs the way it did in her youth.

Marlene and I met shortly after she got this explanation from her other doctor. Once I explained the Keto-Green protocol, she decided to give it a go. She was amazed at the quick results. In the first week she dropped seven pounds and felt more energetic, physically and mentally, than ever. After sixteen days she had lost a total of ten pounds and an inch from her waistline.

Prior to starting the diet, Marlene had trouble sleeping, with frequent awakenings during the night. The reason for this was that her cortisol levels were elevated at night, when they should normally be low. The diet helped restore her body clock so that cortisol would stay in balance—higher during the day to keep her alert, and lower at night to help her sleep. Only a few of her hormones were out of whack, but she got them back in balance by going Keto-Green. Marlene quickly kick-started her metabolism and overcame the hormone changes causing her symptoms.

You can figure out where your imbalances are coming from through testing, along with noting physical symptoms (which I've listed under each hormone in the following sections). We all go through hormonal shifts throughout our lives—caused by puberty, pregnancy, and especially menopause—so paying attention to the subtle signs is key. With the knowledge in this book, you can rebalance your weight-control hormones using the specific diet and exercise strategies I'll provide.

Let's take a look at each of these hormones and how they affect your weight, belly fat, brain, and overall metabolism.

Estrogen

Estrogen creates your curvy feminine shape—your breasts, hips, and even your face. It keeps your skin smooth, tight, and wrinkle-free, and your vagina moist. It is the number-one hormone of womanhood.

Estrogen is also a master regulating hormone that controls energy metabolism in the brain. To do this, it utilizes a network of estrogen receptors throughout a pathway (called the glycolytic pathway) that handles the transport of glucose to the brain. Your brain requires glucose to function, and at an even more basic level, its cells need glucose for survival. Even brief periods of glucose deprivation will result in the death of brain cells. Adequate estrogen levels help feed your brain the glucose it requires to function optimally. With the decline of estrogen, ketones become an optimal substitute.

Along with regulating glucose transport, estrogen supports overall health, helps regulate mitochondrial function, and promotes the generation of ATP (adenosine triphosphate), a storage molecule that provides the energy for many life functions. Mitochondria are like little power plants, supplying energy to the cells in the form of ATP. Mitochondria are vulnerable and can become impaired by various factors our bodies encounter daily, one being oxidative stress—a situation when the body produces more cell-damaging free radicals than our antioxidants can fight off.

When estrogen and other hormones such as progesterone decline during perimenopause and menopause, and cortisol and insulin go up, you enter what I call the state of neuroendocrine vulnerability. This refers to the link between the brain and the endocrine system.

The two are connected through the hypothalamic-pituitary-adrenal (HPA) axis, a complex set of interactions among the brain, pituitary gland, and adrenals that controls metabolism and energy.

With neuroendocrine vulnerability, you're prone to migraines, depression, moodiness, memory loss, and brain fog. It's difficult to make clear decisions or solve problems. Mood drugs like antidepressants won't help either; in fact, they'll ultimately hurt your brain and possibly increase your risk of Alzheimer's disease.

A big part of what's happening in neuroendocrine vulnerability is that the glycolytic pathway is impaired and the brain begins to starve from a lack of glucose. This in turn affects overall cognitive function and may accelerate the risk of Alzheimer's disease and dementia. No wonder the estrogen decline we experience in our forties starts to result in all these unpleasant brain symptoms.

Many scientists believe that perimenopause might provide women a window of time for preventing neuroendocrine vulnerability and enhancing their long-term brain health. During perimenopause, the estrogen receptor network can be greatly influenced, with the potential result being a positive impact on neurological dysfunction or even prevention of age-related neurological diseases.

This has become known as the "window of opportunity" theory: a limited time during which estrogen HRT (hormone replacement therapy) can exert a positive effect on brain function, assuming that a woman's neurological health is not yet compromised in some way.

When I prescribe hormones, I recommend bioidentical hormones, which are identical to the hormones our body produces. Unfortunately, a lot of hormone therapy is initiated by women only after menopause or in early postmenopause—beyond that window of opportunity.

Does this mean estrogen HRT during perimenopause is the only avenue for supporting brain health? What about women who don't wish to or shouldn't take HRT, or who are past that window of opportunity? Is it hopeless for them?

Not at all. When you go Keto-Green, your body enters the fat-burning state of ketosis and produces ketone bodies. As I explained in the introduction, these compounds provide a great fuel source for the brain—an alternative to glucose. In fact, there has been a lot of ongoing research relating to the positive effect of ketones on brain health, dementia, and Alzheimer's disease. Keto-Green provides both the fat-burning benefits and the brain-health benefits associated with ketones and ketosis. Your brain gets the energy it needs—so goodbye brain fog and other symptoms of neuroendocrine vulnerability. You'll think more clearly and make better decisions, including healthy decisions about what to eat.

Let me add that the midlife drop in estrogen also leads to a shift of fat to the midsection. But once you get into ketosis, that belly fat begins to burn right off.

Though as a general rule estrogen is your friend, it's important to understand that there are bad forms of estrogen that can contribute to weight gain. They are called xenoestrogens. These anti-slimming substances enter our bodies through exposure to the chemicals in plastics, food, water, skincare products, the soil, and air. Once there, they mimic natural estrogen, causing a disruption in our natural hormonal balance by affecting hormone communication and signaling. These interactions influence weight negatively and block weight loss. Fortunately, there are foods that detoxify these bad estrogens and eliminate them from the body, and these foods are on the Keto-Green 16 diet.

Signs you may have low estrogen:

✓ You're gaining weight, particularly around your belly, and it's hard to lose it.

✓ Your period gets lighter and more irregular or has disappeared altogether (you've entered menopause).

✓ You have mood swings.

✓ You have trouble sleeping and feel fatigued during the day.

✓ You feel depressed more often.

✓ Your sex drive is low.

✓ Sex is more painful due to vaginal dryness.

✓ Your skin is dryer than usual. Fine lines and wrinkles are emerging on your face.

✓ You experience hot flashes and night sweats.

✓ You have brain fog (poor memory or lack of focus or both).

Progesterone

Progesterone is a neuroprotective hormone vital to brain health. I call it the "calm, cool, collected hormone" because of its positive effect on mood. Like estrogen, progesterone is your friend!

One of progesterone's responsibilities to the brain is to increase an important chemical known as brain-derived neurotrophic factor (BDNF). BDNF preserves the brain's ability to grow and change through the years in response to new challenges, and to resist depression, memory loss, brain shrinkage, and cognitive problems. Progesterone also prevents brain cell death, protects the sheaths around nerves, and reduces the anxiety-provoking effects of glutamate, another type of brain chemical.

The challenge after your thirties is that progesterone begins to decline, and with it goes the ability to fully protect your brain and nerves. Falling progesterone precipitates declining estrogen, which causes a drop in glucose utilization in the female brain. This leads to neuroendocrine vulnerability and may accelerate brain aging.

Low progesterone also causes levels of gamma-aminobutyric acid (GABA) to fall off. GABA is an amino acid and one of the brain's chief calming neurotransmitters. When you're low on GABA, you tend to become more anxious, depressed, and sleep-deprived.

Our bones and connective tissue have receptors (cellular gateways) for progesterone. As the hormone declines with age, these get less progesterone, causing the aching and stiffness that many women feel in their joints.

Signs you may have low progesterone (assuming you are not pregnant):

✓   You're gaining weight, especially around the middle.

✓   You're experiencing headaches and migraines.

✓   You have mood swings, including anxiety and depression.

✓   You're having hot flashes and night sweats.

✓   Your sex drive is low.

✓   You have trouble sleeping and feel fatigued during the day.

✓   Your joints ache or are less flexible.

✓   You have adult-onset acne.

✓   Your menstrual cycle is irregular.

✓   You have brain fog.

Testosterone

Testosterone is often thought of as a male hormone, and that's true, but it is important to both sexes because it protects many vital organs. It is also responsible for boosting libido. From a weight-control perspective, testosterone helps develop muscle and reduce fat, including cellulite.

Age-related declines in testosterone lead to a reduction in calorie-burning muscle tissue for both men and women. Muscles torch calories not just while we work out but when we're resting too, so losing muscle mass means we are burning less fat. Low testosterone also contributes to fat around the waistline.

Signs you may have low testosterone (women):

✓   You're gaining weight.

✓   You're losing muscle tone.

✓   You've lost muscle strength.

✓   Your skin has become thin and dry.

✓   You have trouble sleeping and feel fatigued during the day.

✓   Your sex drive is low.

✓ Sex is more painful due to vaginal dryness.

✓ You've lost bone mass.

✓ Your menstrual cycle is irregular.

✓ You have brain fog.

✓ You feel like you've lost your edge.

DHEA

This acronym stands for dehydroepiandrosterone—that's a hard-to-pronounce mouthful, so no wonder it goes by its initials. DHEA is one of several hormones produced by the adrenal glands, which sit atop your kidneys. The body converts it into estrogen, testosterone, and other less well-known hormones. DHEA also activates receptors on cells that influence how we metabolize and store fat. The peak levels of DHEA are when we are around twenty years old, and from that point on, production starts to go downhill.

In 2004, the National Institutes of Health sponsored a study of DHEA in slightly overweight adults between the ages of sixty-five and seventy-eight. Half supplemented with 50 mg of DHEA daily—a fairly typical dose for men, but very high for women, for whom I typically recommend 5–15 mg—while the other half took a placebo.

Supplementing with DHEA didn't cause any significant weight loss. Participants taking the hormone lost, on average, about two pounds, while those taking the placebo gained a little more than one pound. But, the results for the loss of abdominal fat were more dramatic.

At the end of the six-month study, MRI images revealed that the women taking the hormone had shed about 10 percent of their abdominal fat and the men about 7 percent. That may not seem like much, but certainly anything that reduces abdominal fat merits some attention because belly fat is such a metabolic troublemaker. Fortunately, you can boost this hormone with the help of the right diet.

Signs you may have low DHEA:

✓   You're gaining weight.

✓   You have a hard time developing muscle mass.

✓   Your muscles aren't as strong as they once were (muscle weakness).

✓   You're fatigued during the day.

✓   You've lost your sex drive.

✓   You've been diagnosed with diabetes, osteoporosis, heart disease, or adrenal fatigue.

✓   You are prone to bone fractures.

✓   Your vaginal walls have thinned, and there is little to no lubrication (vaginal atrophy).

✓   You often feel depressed or moody.

✓   You have brain fog.

Insulin

Insulin is one of the three major control hormones, along with cortisol and oxytocin. Insulin affects many other hormones, including estrogen, progesterone, and testosterone. When it is unbalanced, other hormones go out of whack too. Insulin is also a fat-forming hormone responsible for depositing fat on the midsection, hips, and thighs.

Insulin's number one job is to break down glucose in the body and transport it into cells for energy. But as we get older, our bodies can't deal with a lot of carbohydrates. Which means that glucose from carbs you eat—even healthy ones like fruits, whole grains, potatoes, or brown rice—begins to amass in the bloodstream.

In response, the pancreas churns out more and more insulin to help eliminate the excess glucose. But insulin piles up too. There is so much insulin floating around that cells stop paying attention to it—like we might do with the background hum of a refrigerator or the ever-present sight of household clutter. This condition is called insulin resistance. At that point, cells can no longer soak up the extra glucose for fuel. The liver has to deal with it by converting it into fat. Insulin resistance thus causes weight gain, particularly around the waistline.

As you'll see shortly, one clear way to heal insulin resistance is to stop eating sugar, processed carbs, pasta, bread, grains, and starchy vegetables and rely on other forms of energy from your diet. My combination of keto and alkaline eating helps regulate insulin and reverse insulin resistance in one important way: It shifts you into ketosis, and that means fat-burning. This restores your body to an insulin-sensitive state, in which cells begin to notice insulin and again allow it to usher glucose into cells for energy.

Insulin also plays an important role in brain function, especially in learning and memory. Research has found that cognitively healthy individuals will display mental and intellectual deficits when their insulin function is reduced.

There is also an association between a high-glycemic diet (characterized by a lot of simple carbohydrates and sugars) and a greater incidence of a condition called cerebral amyloid burden, observed in people with Alzheimer's disease. This happens when corrupted proteins called amyloids gang up in the brain, forming plaques that kill brain cells. Amyloid deposits are also closely linked to the development of type 2 diabetes.

Going Keto-Green helps your body become more insulin sensitive, and possibly helps protect against this type of brain damage. Another benefit of improved insulin sensitivity (above and beyond a healthy brain and weight loss) is less frequent hot flashes.

Signs you may be insulin-resistant:

✓ You're gaining weight, including around your midsection.

✓ You're having night sweats and hot flashes.

✓ You're fatigued during the day.

✓   Your blood sugar tends to stay elevated.

✓   You've been diagnosed with high blood pressure and high cholesterol.

✓   You often feel hungry, even after a meal, or experience hypoglycemic symptoms.

✓   You crave sugar and processed carbs.

✓   You urinate more often.

✓   You feel more thirsty than usual.

✓   You get sick or have infections more often.

Glucagon

Something else happens when you restrict carbs and replace them with clean proteins and plenty of fresh, non-starchy vegetables: You stimulate the production of glucagon, a hormone that helps burn body fat (unlike insulin, which helps the body store fat). These two hormones act like a chemical seesaw. As levels of insulin go up, glucagon production goes down. As levels of glucagon rise, insulin production drops.

Remember that if a meal generates more glucose than you can use at the moment, the pancreas produces insulin to get the excess out of your bloodstream. Later, as blood sugar declines and insulin drops, glucagon is released from the liver, causing the body to utilize alternative energy sources (such as fat stores) in the absence of glucose.

Everything hums along nicely as long as insulin and glucagon stay in a dynamic balance. But if we continually eat more carbs than we can burn off, insulin gets the upper hand, and the pounds start piling on.

Eating healthy protein (lean meat, fish, nuts, and seeds) stimulates the release of glucagon. It is then able to unlock fat stores, keep blood sugar steady between meals, and prevent the body from producing too much insulin—which means less fat storage. It's rare for someone to make too little glucagon.

Adiponectin

You've probably never heard of adiponectin, so let me introduce you. Produced by fat cells, adiponectin acts in the brain to help you lose weight and protect against gaining belly fat. Specifically, this hormone works through the melanocortin pathway in the brain—a system that affects many processes in the body, including the urge to eat, pigment formation in our skin, inflammation, energy levels, and sex drive.

Adiponectin encourages greater use of glucose by your muscles. It also decreases the production of glucose by your liver, and promotes the use of fat stores for energy. All this helps you become more insulin sensitive—which makes it easier to control your weight.

There's more too. Adiponectin may fight weight-loss plateaus and raise your metabolic rate without affecting appetite.

You'd think that someone who is very overweight would produce a lot of this fat-burning hormone, but this isn't so. If you have a lot of fat on your body, including belly fat, less adiponectin is produced, and your blood glucose levels stay high, promoting insulin resistance. As you lose weight, your body churns out more fat-burning adiponectin.

There are specific foods that help raise adiponectin in the body, including good fats such as avocados and olives, spices like turmeric, and fibrous veggies—foods that are part of the Keto-Green 16 plan.

Signs that you may be low in adiponectin:

✓ You struggle with obesity.

✓ Your doctor feels your visceral fat is excessive.

✓ You've been diagnosed with insulin resistance.

✓ Your annual blood test reveals markers for inflammation.

Cortisol

Here's a hormone I'm sure you've heard of, especially if you've read my first book, *The Hormone Fix*. Cortisol is the key stress hormone and, essentially, a lifesaver. It is an immediate responder in times of danger and stress. If you find yourself in a threatening situation—needing to suddenly swerve out of the way of another car in traffic, for instance—your adrenal glands pour out cortisol. Cortisol boosts the amount of blood sugar available for fuel and revs up your heart rate so you can fight off or escape a threat, or otherwise deal with the stress.

Although cortisol mobilizes the body to deal with danger and stress, if it stays elevated in the body for too long, usually due to chronic, unresolved stress, it becomes a troublemaker. When it hangs around too long, cortisol can trigger a fat-storing enzyme in visceral fat cells, causing many of us to put on more belly fat. Belly fat cells have four times as many cortisol receptors as regular fat cells. This means that they attract more fat-storing cortisol, with the consequence of more fat around the waist.

Lingering cortisol also raises your blood sugar levels and keeps them high. This leads to insulin resistance. As a result of elevated glucose levels, the brain sends out hunger signals that can cause overeating.

Further, consistently raised levels of cortisol will cause memory issues, high blood pressure, insomnia, and immune system suppression. When the adrenals are overworked and churning out too much cortisol, this impedes their ability to produce other protective hormones (such as progesterone, pregnenolone, and DHEA).

Switching to more alkaline foods and pursuing certain stress-management lifestyle habits curtail levels of cortisol, which is one reason that both actions help you lose body fat and feel more mentally alive. There is a definite and positive connection between following an alkaline diet and a less-stressed lifestyle—and therefore lowering cortisol and burning fat.

Signs you may have elevated cortisol:

✓ You're gaining weight, mostly around the midsection and upper back.

✓ You have adult-onset acne.

✓ Your skin is thinning and bruises easily.

✓ You have trouble sleeping at night.

✓ You're tired during the day.

✓ Your muscles aren't as strong as they once were (muscle weakness).

✓ You feel irritable.

✓ You have frequent headaches.

✓ You have difficulty concentrating.

✓ You've been diagnosed with high blood pressure.

Oxytocin

Meet my favorite hormone, oxytocin. It's the hormone of love, bonding, and connection. It is released during sex, orgasms, cuddling, childbirth, and breastfeeding.

But what does oxytocin have to do with weight control? Plenty, it turns out. For one thing, it counters the surge of cortisol, which, as we've just learned, can be a belly-fat promoter.

Another way oxytocin works is by limiting the amount of food that we eat. It does this by speeding up the satiety process, making us feel full faster. Also, it works through brain areas that are associated with the pleasure of eating, decreasing our urge to eat purely for pleasure. Oxytocin, in other words, appears to make food seem less rewarding, so we're less apt to reach for that second slice of cheesecake.

What's more, oxytocin improves insulin sensitivity and encourages the body to use fat as fuel.

Signs you may be running low on oxytocin:

✓ You're gaining weight.

✓ You're suffering indigestion.

✓ You feel pessimistic.

✓ Your sex life has become mechanical.

✓   You're less affectionate.

✓   You're more irritable than usual.

Thyroid

Hidden inside the base of your neck, in front of your windpipe, is the tiny butterfly-shaped thyroid gland—the body's metabolism master. Like the drummer in a rock band, the thyroid gland establishes the body's rhythms. It does this by releasing two hormones—T3 and T4—that regulate heartbeat, body temperature, the rate at which your body burns calories, and more.

Many patients come to me dealing with thyroid disease, usually low or underactive thyroid. I've been there myself. Several years ago, after I'd had to deal with flooding in the aftermath of two separate hurricanes in a year and live with toxic black mold issues, my own levels of TSH (thyroid-stimulating hormone) skyrocketed to over 5.4. A high TSH concentration indicates an underactive thyroid that isn't secreting enough hormones. But when I got back on my Keto-Green diet, it reduced to a beautiful number, 0.77, which is in the optimal range of 0.4 to 2.0.

The thyroid can cause big health problems when it misfires—far bigger than anyone until lately ever realized. I want to assure you, however, that most thyroid problems can be corrected with simple changes in your lifestyle, particularly a low-carb, alkaline diet like mine.

An example is Tina, a fifty-six-year-old woman who followed my Keto-Green eating plan and lifestyle program for about eight months. Her T3 level increased from 2.8 to 2.9, and her TSH decreased from 2.9 to 1.94, which is more optimal. She felt great too.

In a survey of more than five hundred women following my dietary advice, 95 percent felt that their energy levels had soared. Many women who had their thyroid tested saw their numbers improve across the board. That's great, since lower T3 levels have actually been associated with some good things, such as preserved muscle mass (for greater fat burning) and even a longer life span. As you'll soon see, my diet includes thyroid-protective foods, including white fish and Brazil nuts.

Signs you may have an underactive thyroid:

✓ You've started gaining weight for no apparent reason.

✓ You feel exhausted and sluggish.

✓ You suffer gas, bloating, and abdominal cramps with foods you've eaten for years with no problems.

✓ You feel irritable, depressed, or moody.

✓ You often feel cold.

✓ Your hair is thinning.

Of special note: Tests for thyroid function often miss the mark because these tests typically focus on detecting levels of TSH only. I recommend getting a full thyroid profile that includes TSH, free T4, free T3, reverse T3, thyroid peroxidase antibodies, and anti-thyroglobulin antibodies. (See dranna.com/KetoGreenBook.)

Growth Hormone (GH)

Produced by the pituitary gland, growth hormone determines our ultimate size and height. The body requires this hormone for metabolism and to ensure normal growth and development, especially during childhood.

Growth hormone also tones and firms muscles, strengthens our bones, and protects our organs. What's more, it prevents obesity, decreases fat, and firms our thighs, hips, and stomach muscles. Growth hormone is commonly considered an anti-aging hormone because it helps us stay young-looking.

By the time we reach age seventy, our growth hormone levels have fallen by about 40 percent, resulting in a 30 percent reduction in muscle strength. When we have too little growth hormone, our fat cells don't hear the brain's signal to burn fat for energy. Studies show that adults who lack enough growth hormone often have a lot of body fat, especially around the trunk.

A nutrition plan sufficient in protein like my Keto-Green 16 enhances the effectiveness of growth hormone by supplying the amino acids that the hormone requires to work in muscles, skin, bones, and other organs. Supplemental amino acids such as lysine act as "secretogogues" that provide the natural release of GH.

High-intensity interval training (HIIT) on a regular basis also increases growth hormone. Sleep is key too. During the night, your pituitary gland secretes growth hormone, which stimulates fat cells to release energy to repair the body's tissues.

Signs you may be low in growth hormone:

✓ You lack muscle density.

✓ You've lost muscle strength.

✓ You carry fat on your hips, thighs, and tummy.

✓ You have cellulite.

✓ You've lost interest in sex.

✓ You feel depressed.

✓ Your skin is dry and thin.

✓ You're tired during the day.

✓ You have brain fog.

✓ You've been diagnosed with insulin resistance, elevated triglycerides, or high LDL cholesterol.

Leptin

By now you may have heard of the hormone leptin. Secreted by fat cells, leptin is nicknamed the "satiety hormone" because it sends a message to your brain and body that you are full, so you don't need to eat anymore, and that it's time to start burning calories.

Leptin is interconnected with the hypothalamus, the part of the brain that regulates food intake, energy expenditure, and glucose and fat metabolism. When you lose weight, your fat stores shrink and therefore produce less leptin. The hypothalamus thinks your body might be starving, so it sends out signals to eat more and expend less energy. Although this response is a normal defense mechanism, it becomes difficult to maintain weight loss unless you get leptin back in balance. How do you bring it back into balance? With the right foods.

In some people, the brain receptors responsible for processing leptin just don't function the way they should. A possible explanation is that these people produce too much leptin. The excess overloads their brain receptors, making them less sensitive to leptin. When this happens, the brain eventually stops hearing the messages telling it to stop eating. It is like the begging dog at the dinner table—you ignore it and just keep eating your meal, not paying any attention (you know what I mean). This is called leptin resistance.

The Keto-Green 16 plan prevents leptin resistance and therefore reduces cravings. Plus the plan provides lots of nutrients that help normalize leptin, including taurine (an essential amino acid found in meat, chicken, and fish) and vitamin A (available from fish).

Signs that you may be leptin-resistant:

✓ You gain weight quickly.

✓ You carry a lot of weight around your waist.

✓ You have a tough time losing weight.

✓ You're constantly hungry.

✓ You frequently have cravings for certain foods.

Ghrelin

Your stomach is starting to rumble. Or maybe you've got a headache because you haven't had a meal yet. In both cases, your body is sending a clear signal: Give me food, right now!

These heavy-duty hunger signals may not be due to weak willpower. A hormone named ghrelin may be responsible. Identified in 1999, ghrelin is produced in your stomach. It travels through your bloodstream and to your brain, where it announces: "It's time to eat!"

The higher your levels of ghrelin, the hungrier you'll be. The lower your levels, the fuller you'll feel. So if you want to lose weight, lowering your ghrelin levels is helpful. You can do this easily through diet.

A benefit of a keto diet is that it can suppress your appetite, partly by stabilizing both ghrelin and leptin. A keto diet supplies plenty of fat and protein, two macronutrients that increase fullness and reduce hunger.

The main sign that your ghrelin levels may be too high is constant hunger.

HORMONE TESTING

The level of most of these hormones in your system can be easily tested. The purpose of testing is to check your hormone levels to see whether or not they are in the proper range. Here are two hormone panels I recommend:

TEST PANEL	WHAT IT INCLUDES	HOW IT'S DONE
Comprehensive metabolic and hormone panel	Complete blood count (CBC), complete metabolic panel, cortisol, DHEA-S (if not done separately), total estrogens, estradiol, progesterone, testosterone (free and total), hemoglobin A1c (HbA1c), hsC-reactive protein (hsCRP), fractionated blood lipids, red blood cell magnesium, vitamin D, and thyroid hormones (free T4, free T3, TSH, reverse T3 and thyroid antibodies, among others). Additional tests, depending on individual needs, might include a ferritin and iron panel, IGF-1, adiponectin, melatonin, red blood count, zinc, and estrogen detoxification panel.	Blood test
Adrenal stress index	This test gives a more comprehensive understanding of adrenal hormone balance by assessing cortisol and DHEA throughout the day. It is an ideal evaluation for those under chronic stress with known or suspected endocrine abnormalities. It tests for six different hormones and immune markers that may be affected by chronic stress and stress-related conditions.	Saliva test

I also invite you to look at my Hormonal Review of Symptoms Checklist, which is on my website, dranna.com/KetoGreenBook. It will provide insight into any hormonal deficiencies you might have and takes only minutes to complete.

Keto-Green 16 maximizes every one of these hormones for rapid fat loss, as long as you stick to the plan. And, trust me, you can, especially because you'll see results daily! It doesn't matter how often you have failed in the past; your past dieting experiences do not forecast your future. What matters now is that you stay upbeat and positive, and believe in yourself and the power of this program. Your appearance, your self-confidence, your happiness, and your health are worth it.

Chapter 2

Just Give Me 16 Days

. . . .

You're about to start the best and easiest way to burn fat, trim your waistline, balance hormones, and boost your energy. What you'll do over the next sixteen days will rapidly change the way you look and feel, while building a foundation of disease prevention for the rest of your life.

That's a big promise, I know! Proof that it works: In August and September 2019, I conducted two studies with forty-three women and several men on the Keto-Green 16 diet. In the first study, participants (ages forty-nine to seventy-one) lost up to eleven pounds, trimmed one to two inches off their waistlines, and improved their diastolic blood pressure (the bottom number, which describes the pressure on the arteries between heartbeats).

The participants also filled out a Medical Symptom Toxicity Questionnaire before and after the sixteen-day program. This assessment looks into issues such as digestion, presence of headaches or brain fog, skin health, eating behavior, eyes, energy levels, and more. On average, the participants had major drops in their score, meaning that their bodies had started functioning more normally and at a higher level of health.

Results were similar for the second study, with a few differences.

The subjects in this study ranged from fifty-one to seventy-five years old and were 90 percent women. My primary focus was pounds lost and inches lost around the waist. The average weight loss among participants was 5.5 pounds in sixteen days. Some people lost twelve to thirteen pounds during the study! As for belly fat, the average number of inches shaved from the midsection was 1.14 inches, with some participants losing as much as 2.2 inches. With a similar outcome, you might be able to drop a size or two in sixteen days!

How I Developed This Diet

My journey into the world of nutritional medicine really began from a serious hormone imbalance I experienced after my toddler son died in a tragic accident. His death left me bereft, grieving, traumatized, and broken in so many ways. Eventually I had to pull my life and my family back together, despite suffering from lingering PTSD. I delved into the underlying effects of trauma in my book *The Hormone Fix,* as well as many aspects of my own healing journey through grief and trauma.

There was so much of my life that was out of control. I was devastated physically, mentally, emotionally, and spiritually. To make things worse, I was told that I'd never be able to have another child because I was infertile. I tried infertility drugs, but they all failed.

My doctor's bag was empty!

So I took a sabbatical and traveled around the world on a healing trek, looking and praying for answers. What I discovered helped me in so many ways, including reversing my early menopause (brought on by the PTSD) and then allowing me to conceive a child at age forty-one.

By the end of the trip, my doctor's bag was full! I had learned about diet, herbs, spirituality, and other healing tools. As a result, I restored myself. I lost more than eighty pounds. I renewed my hair, skin, and vitality. And best of all, I came back reinvigorated to help thousands of women like myself.

I still had struggles, though. PTSD simmered under the surface of my soul. My marriage crumbled and I got a divorce. I was burned out. Then, when I was forty-eight, twenty pounds piled back on my body—seemingly overnight. I was sick of the constant weight battles and had enough. I knew I had to do something fast.

Keto On!

I felt that a ketogenic diet might work for me because it takes pounds off rather quickly and it has positive effects on brain health and clear thinking—which I needed desperately as a single mom charged with supporting my family.

A conventional ketogenic diet is one that is very low in carbs, high in fats, and moderate in protein. It burns fat very efficiently, but there are side effects, such as "keto flu," which makes you feel strange, like you have the real flu. Its symptoms include fatigue, diarrhea, nausea, body aches, and headaches. Although a keto diet can foster clear thinking, it can also make you feel moody and mentally unstable—what I call "keto craziness"—as the brain shifts from using glucose to an alternative source of energy (ketone bodies). I experienced all of this, and I felt terrible—not what I needed!

While I was trying to figure out what was wrong with me, I tested my urine using simple pH strips you can get at any pharmacy. My own test showed that I was highly acidic. That was an aha moment. When the body gets too acidic, we are much more vulnerable to getting sick. No wonder I felt so terrible on a keto diet.

I decided to further change my eating habits to make my body more alkaline. I began eating more greens and drinking bone broth. Within days of making these changes, I felt more energetic. My mind was even more clear and focused. The weight started peeling off, and I lost those twenty pounds in no time. I felt great.

I then undertook some research and found a journal article published in 1924 in the *Biochemical Journal* from the Biochemical Laboratory in Cambridge, England. It evaluated a ketogenic diet with alkalinity and implied that the combination could be very beneficial and therapeutic.

I dug into the science even more and learned that if you stay on a pure keto diet too long, your body may become acidic, creating chronic inflammation that forces your body to hold on to its fat stores. This is especially true for women—I've seen this play out numerous times among my female patients. (It does not happen as much with men, most likely because they have ten times more testosterone than we do, thus cooling the inflammation.) For women, getting alkaline is a key factor in undoing that inflammation and all its negative effects.

Because this keto-alkaline approach that I created worked so well for me, I began putting clients on it via my online Magic Menopause programs. The participants began breezing through menopause and its symptoms. They lost weight, reached their happy weight, rejuvenated their appearance, felt more energetic and healthy, and balanced their hormones. Thousands of women have now experienced these amazing results.

As for me, I'm fifty-three with four daughters, the youngest of whom is eleven years old, and I've never felt better, thanks to adding alkaline foods and an alkaline lifestyle to a healthy keto diet. I feel fabulous, physically and mentally, and I want that for you too. The Keto-Green 16 diet is the next right step for you.

The Keto-Green Difference: An Overview

Some general background first. The Keto-Green 16 diet is low-carb. In fact, I advise that you restrict your carbohydrate intake to no more than 40 grams a day. As we get older, we simply cannot process carbohydrates like we did in our youth. Carbs tend to impair insulin's job of processing fuel properly—that's the insulin resistance I explained in Chapter 1 (see page 14). As a result, the body stores more fat than usual, especially around the belly. Reduce carbs, and you prevent insulin resistance and the fat accumulation that comes with it.

Unlike conventional keto diets, my plan is a super-healthy approach that focuses on "keto-clean" foods and de-emphasizes "keto-dirty" foods. Keto-clean foods are whole, unprocessed foods that are high in fiber and low in carbs but are still packed with other nutrients. Examples are high-fiber veggies, green leafy vegetables, nuts and seeds, avocados, coconut oil, and ghee. Dirty-keto foods are items like bacon grease, pork rinds, and processed cheeses. Even low-carb packaged convenience foods such as protein bars and other snacks count as dirty keto and are to be avoided.

My diet is high in fat, but it focuses on the right fats, such as olive oil, olives, avocados, coconut oil, nuts, and seeds. They taste delicious and make your food more palatable. Plus they're filling.

Keto-Green 16 is moderate in protein, preferably unprocessed, organic, and grass-fed beef, organic and free-range poultry, wild-caught fish, and vegetarian protein sources. Protein is a great metabolism booster. Research has found that people who eat more and better-quality protein have much less belly fat and are less prone to gaining it.

The real all-stars of this diet are alkalinizing vegetables, particularly leafy greens like spinach, lettuce, kale, chard, beet greens, mustard greens, collard greens, and sprouts. Cruciferous veggies like cabbage, broccoli, Brussels sprouts, and cauliflower also play starring roles. These are just a few of the many satisfying veggies you can eat. They are very low in carbs and high in nutrients, vitamins, and antioxidants. And they'll help keep your body alkaline— a healthy internal state of well-being and metabolic efficiency. You'll start dropping weight like crazy and feel on top of your game.

Very important: You'll soon discover that the Keto-Green 16 plan layers in intermittent fasting, a super-easy lose-fat strategy. We practice it already without realizing it. It's called sleeping! On my plan, it involves going without food from dinner one day to a later breakfast the next day—a period of sixteen hours. You'll discover that intermittent fasting on this plan is a real game-changer, one that you'll want in your weight-control toolbox for the rest of your life.

And one more thing. I believe in "feasting" meals too. This is a healthy and fun carb-up day, typically every seven to ten days. It keeps our bodies metabolically flexible. Good choices for these "feasts" are sweet potatoes and fresh fruit; my guilty pleasure is dark chocolate. Also, this practice keeps us from feeling deprived and better able to stay on track 90 percent of the time.

Keto Explained

When you restrict carbohydrates on a keto diet, you reduce the production of glucose and therefore reduce the production of insulin. Your body looks around for something other than glucose to burn for energy. What does it burn? Stored fat! A ketogenic diet works by keeping the body's carbohydrate stores almost empty. This stimulates the production of glucagon, which unlocks your fat stores. Your body starts burning its own fat for energy, helping you lose weight quickly. It will also burn the fat you're eating in your diet.

Keto dieting is definitely an effective way to lose weight. A 2018 report out of Framingham State University found that after five months on a keto diet, overweight adults burned about 250 more calories daily than people who followed a high-carb, low-fat diet. This study, published in the *British Medical Journal*, also showed that dieters on a keto-type diet had increased energy expenditure—aka a faster metabolism—than those on higher carb diets. Don't be surprised if you quickly feel much more energetic on Keto-Green 16!

When your body doesn't have carbs, it goes into a metabolic state called ketosis. In ketosis, your body gets its energy from ketone bodies in your blood. Ketone bodies (ketones for short) are molecules produced from the breakdown of fat. After about three days without carbs, most of your carbohydrate stores will be depleted. Your body goes into a hyper-fat-burning mode and produces ketone bodies for fuel instead of glucose.

As you continue to eat this way, you become "fat-adapted," which means that your body primarily uses fat as energy instead of glucose. Normally our bodies run on a fuel mix of glucose and fat, but in a non-fat-adapted state, the body taps into glucose first. Once you are fat-adapted, though, your body is in a continual state of fat-burning. It doesn't even miss the glucose it used to get from carbs.

Ketones are especially critical for the brain. Most of your body, including your muscles, can run on fat, but the brain can only refuel on either ketones or glucose. A keto diet increases the number of mitochondria—the energy factories—of brain cells and all other cells of the body. Those mitochondria prefer ketones as fuel. This probably accounts for the feelings of mental clarity and energy you'll experience on this diet, as well as a faster metabolic rate. In fact, I draw the analogy that glucose is to ketones as gasoline is to jet fuel—ketones are a supercharged form of brain fuel.

A keto diet optimizes blood sugar and insulin levels. One study among people with type 2 diabetes found such dramatic glucose improvements that they could stop taking or reduce their diabetes medications. (*Please never reduce or discontinue any medication without your doctor's approval.*) Among its other duties, insulin is designed to store fat, so when insulin levels go down, fat-burning goes up.

One of the other benefits you'll notice from being in ketosis is less hunger. You'll feel fuller for longer, partly because of the good fats and clean proteins you'll be eating, but also because ketosis changes your levels of the hunger hormones ghrelin and leptin. Specifically, the diet decreases hunger-creating ghrelin and increases hunger-suppressing leptin, so you feel more satisfied and have fewer cravings.

Not only does ketosis help you tame hunger, burn overall fat, and encourage weight loss, but a study published in the journal *Endocrine* found that the diet targets inflammatory visceral (belly) fat in particular. Remember, visceral fat is considered a risk factor for heart disease, cancer, and diabetes because it wraps around key organs and leaks toxins into them.

A ketogenic diet can sometimes be difficult to stick with, but here's what I've seen among my patients: Once they get into the swing of things and see results, keto becomes much easier. They know what foods to eat and avoid, their cravings and hunger vanish, and they start dropping pounds and feeling fabulous. Sometimes people even ask them if they've "had some work done."

Alkalinity, Explained

In simple terms, an alkaline diet is a way of eating that emphasizes non-acidifying foods over acidifying ones. You make your food choices around those that lower the acid levels in your body and increase its alkalinity. My Keto-Green 16 plan emphasizes many healthy, alkalinizing foods. I discuss acidity versus alkalinity extensively on my website, dranna.com, so be sure to check it out for extra credit.

In a substantial amount of research, a more optimal alkaline pH status in the body has been found to:

- Support bone health and lean muscle mass

- Reduce pain and inflammation

- Lower risk of disease (cardiovascular disease, hypertension, insulin resistance, diabetes, and metabolic disorders)

- Support the healthy balance of electrolyte levels our bodies require for quality sleep, circadian rhythm control, and cortisol management

- Help the body burn fat

So what exactly does pH mean? It stands for the power of hydrogen or the total hydrogen ion concentration in a solution. PH levels are expressed on a scale from 1 to 14 to specify how acidic or alkaline a water-based solution is. Higher pH numbers are alkaline (also referred to as base) and lower numbers are acidic (acid). A pH of 7 is generally considered neutral.

The human body works hard around the clock to maintain a slightly alkaline pH level in the blood, and to do so it must clear out any excess acid. Your body has a precise mechanism for maintaining its blood acid-base balance, and the mechanism ensures that the pH of blood doesn't shift much at all. It is tightly controlled by the kidneys and lungs to stay at around 7.4. This is critical for human life, because even a small variation in blood pH is life-threatening. This tight regulation declines with age, and there can be an increase in metabolic acidosis because most modern diets are acidic. That's another reason why eating alkaline is even more important as we get older.

While the blood pH stays in a very small range, the rest of your body varies in pH level. Your stomach, for example, is very acidic, typically maintaining a pH of less than 3.0 so that it can fully break down the food you eat and kill ingested pathogens. The pH of your vagina is 3.8–4.4, which is protective and kills off unwanted bacteria, but this pH increases as we age. The skin has a pH below 5. By contrast, the pH of the intestines and pancreas is 8.0. Most cells work best when they are on the alkaline side. The pH of urine, however, fluctuates and serves as a window on what is happening at the cellular and hormonal levels. Ideally, it is good to see the pH of urine at about 7.

PH levels are not just about what we eat but also about how we live. After intense exercise, we expect our pH to be more acidic; after a relaxing day in nature, it will likely be more alkaline. Stress and the resultant elevated cortisol are highly acid-promoting. Every time I walk on the beach in the morning and test my alkalinity afterward, I find that I easily stay alkaline all day. When you discover this for yourself, it will be a huge aha moment.

Current research shows that eating alkaline-forming foods supports the body's natural pH balancing act. Foods on the alkaline end of the scale include vegetables (particularly greens), fermented vegetables (like sauerkraut and kimchi), low-glycemic, low-sugar fruits, and various healthy fats. If you eat enough alkaline-forming foods, your body has better access to vital minerals such as calcium, phosphorus, and magnesium—all of which help improve hormone balance.

As for weight loss, an alkaline diet assists the body in burning fat. First, alkalinity (along with a low-carb diet) decreases levels of cortisol, a hormone responsible for belly fat. When you burn fat, the body releases toxins. Alkaline foods also support detoxification and help usher toxins from the body.

Second, an alkaline diet helps you work out more intensely. Researchers at Saint Louis University have found that alkaline diets improved physical fitness of individuals in comparison to acidic diets. Improving your exercise performance can translate into greater weight loss and more energy.

Third, an alkaline diet protects muscle, the most metabolically active tissue in the body. With more muscle, you burn more calories, even at rest. A study looking at a diet rich in potassium and magnesium (ample in fruits and vegetables), as well as a reduced acid load, found that such a diet preserved muscle in women. The researchers noted: "Although protein is important for maintenance of muscle mass, eating fruits and vegetables that supply adequate amounts of potassium and magnesium are also relevant. The results suggest a potential role for diet in the prevention of muscle loss."

To reduce acid load, you'll want to watch out for acid-forming foods. These include sugar, processed foods, breads, pastas, grains, starchy vegetables, artificial sweeteners, sodas, many meats, and alcohol. They stress your digestive system and cause weight gain, a bloated and fatter belly, sluggish thinking, and tiredness. There are a couple of reasons for this that have been validated by science.

First, there is now increasing evidence to suggest that an acidic diet may be independently associated with the risk of developing type 2 diabetes. A diet with a high acid load can reduce pH toward the lower end of the normal range, which may in turn lead to the development of insulin resistance (a precursor to type 2 diabetes). Conversely, reducing dietary acid load with an alkaline diet may be protective and prevent type 2 diabetes, according to a 2016 diet published in *Biochimie*.

Second, as a study published in 2016 in *Osteoporosis International* reported, an acidic diet can accelerate the loss of muscle tissue, especially in women age sixty and older. We do not want to lose muscle with age! Muscle loss slows down metabolism and makes us look older. We need muscles to burn calories, stay mobile, and be vibrant. The researchers further stated that "an alkaline diet may be beneficial for preserving total lean mass in senior women, especially in those with low protein intake."

Many of us eat a more acidic diet due to our unhealthy food choices (processed foods in particular), but even those who eat healthfully may be unaware of the very different mineral profiles that our foods today have versus what our ancestors ate. Today's farming practices and mineral-poor soils, coupled with the large amount of toxins that foods are now exposed to (including pesticides, antibiotics, and hormones), impact the acidic effects of much of what people eat. In a typical Western diet, there has been a significant increase in sodium and a decrease in potassium, for example. In fact, the ratio of potassium to sodium has reversed and changed dramatically: It used to be 10 to 1, but now in the typical Western diet it is 1 to 3! These changes can impact many of our body's most important processes.

I am not saying we need to completely avoid acidic foods. We need a balance of healthy (organic, grass-fed, and so forth) acidic foods in our diet. The important thing for your best health is the ratio of alkaline to acid in what is on your dinner plate. You need to be looking at the net effect of your diet on your acid-base balance. You can accomplish this using the 80/20 rule. Consume a diet that is 80 percent alkaline (a lot of veggies) and 20 percent acidic (protein and healthy fats). In my women's restorative health programs, we talk about visualizing an actual plate with the healthiest proportion of proteins, healthy carbs (veggies), and healthy fats. (See pages 82 and 83 for ideal Keto-Green 16 plates.)

Also, go organic for higher mineral content and fewer toxins. Non-organic options are likely grown in mineral-depleted soils that are also exposed to toxins. Organic foods optimize your alkalinity.

Keto versus Keto-Green

I am often asked to explain the difference between a keto diet and my Keto-Green plan. For a simplified answer, see the following chart.

THE DIFFERENCES BETWEEN THE KETO DIET AND THE KETO-GREEN 16 DIET	
KETOGENIC DIET	**MY KETO-GREEN DIET**
Favors many acidic foods such as meats	Favors alkaline foods such as green leafy vegetables and other low-calorie veggies
Allows more acidic fats like butter and bacon	Focuses on more alkaline fats like avocado, nuts, and olive oil
Is based on the ratio of eating 60 to 75 percent of your daily calories from fat, 5 to 10 percent of your calories from carbs, and 15 to 30 percent of your daily calories from protein	Is based visually on a plate filled with the following ratio: about 80 percent alkaline foods (with a ton of veggies) and 20 percent acidic with protein-and-healthy-fat-rich meats. It is also based on eating 55 to 75 percent of your daily calories from fat, 5 to 15 percent from carbs, and 15 to 25 percent from protein.
Limits fruits to berries	Allows a larger variety of low-sugar fruits for greater alkalinity
Has potential side effects such as dehydration, nausea, and other issues stemming from eating too many acid-forming foods	Prevents these side effects by incorporating plenty of plant-based fiber-rich alkaline foods
Can build up acidic toxicity in cells	Has a natural detoxifying effect on the body, thanks to the inclusion of vegetables such as broccoli, cauliflower, sprouts, and cabbage—all of which help eliminate the buildup of acidity in your body
Tests urine ketones only	Tests urine ketones *and* alkalinity (pH) with my special Keto-pH test strips, available at dranna.com

Test, Don't Guess: Measuring Ketosis and Alkalinity

To ensure you're on target to experience all of the wonderful benefits of this diet, it's going to be important to measure your levels of ketosis and alkalinity by testing your urine throughout the day (every time you go to the bathroom), using special test strips. In fact, I encourage you to do this through the entire sixteen days. You'll gain valuable information on how well you're burning fat, as well as your alkaline status, and the feedback is motivating. When I've asked an audience of keto dieters if they've been testing for ketones, typically fewer than 10 percent raise their hands.

You can purchase ketone test strips and alkaline test strips in any pharmacy, or you can use my dual-purpose test strips available at dranna.com. They measure ketosis and alkalinity on the same strip and are much handier than using two different strips. Whatever test you use, the results are rapidly expressed as a color change. The pinker the strip, the higher your level of ketosis; the greener the strip, the more alkaline your body. Whatever pH paper or strips you buy will come accompanied by a color chart to compare your results to, so judge your results by that.

How to use my dual-purpose strips:

1. Hold the strip away from the little test pads.

2. Pass the strip in your urine stream or dip it in a urine-filled cup.

3. Set the strip flat on absorbent paper.

4. After forty seconds, match the ketone test pad to the ketone color chart. You want to see pink.

5. After sixty seconds, match the alkaline test pad to the alkaline color chart. You want to have a pH of at least 7; anything less is acidic.

Throughout this book, I'll give you tips on how to get alkaline and stay there, plus how to maintain ketosis over the next sixteen days.

Measuring Your Glucose Levels

In early 2019, I decided to learn how different foods and beverages affected my glucose levels. What raises my blood sugar? What keeps it steady? Rising glucose means more insulin is being churned out—a factor that might impede my fat-burning ability.

I purchased a device called the Freestyle Libre. It is a continuous glucose monitoring system consisting of a handheld reader about the size of a cellphone (or you can obtain the readings from a smartphone with an app) and a sensor worn on the back of your upper arm. The sensor has a thin, flexible filament that inserts painlessly just under the skin. It makes contact with a thin layer of fluid that surrounds the cells of the tissues below your skin, in order to measure glucose every minute. The sensors last two weeks and store up to eight hours of data, displaying it on a graph so you can see if your blood sugar is on an upward or downward trend. It is a great tool for people with diabetes because the readings help them adjust their insulin dose or food intake accordingly.

What I discovered was interesting. Coffee raised my glucose levels—which it does in some caffeine-sensitive people. But low-sugar red wine did not—which is good because I enjoy a nice glass of robust red wine every now and then. On the other hand, I had a sugary cocktail at a party one time, and my blood sugar registered at 220 (normal is around 88).

I also discovered that if I start my day with stressful thoughts, as opposed to positive morning meditation and prayer, my blood sugar shoots up 30 or more points. Once when I was delivering a keynote speech, even though I was fasting, my glucose reading was in the 150s for thirty minutes; another time, when I was doing an intense boxing routine daily, my blood sugar zoomed to 190 even though I was fasting! This makes sense—cortisol and stress increase the release of glucose to help the body function optimally—but this fascinates me.

Monitoring your own glucose with the Freestyle Libre device is optional and not required to get great results on this diet. It is part of the self-discovery detective work I recommend, however. Knowing which foods spike your blood sugar can be helpful when trying to eliminate stubborn fat. Additionally, it is important to see how quickly your blood sugar returns to normal. Ideally, it should take one to two hours to go from spike to recovery. If your blood sugar stays high, it's important to see your physician in order to find out what's going on with your health.

Abigail, one of the women in my study, lost eight pounds in the first six days of the study. She also decided to use the Libre to monitor her glucose. Based on her Libre data, her fasting blood sugar remained in the 80s (very healthy) during the study, and her HbA1c—which measures a person's average level of blood sugar over the past two to three months—dropped to a healthy 5.4 from 6.0 in thirty days. She told me it had not been that optimal in years. And Abigail reported, "More importantly for me, my brain is really clear and I have so much energy."

The Freestyle Libre is a great tool for additional feedback on how the diet is working for you. You can purchase it over the counter for approximately $40, but in some places you may have to ask your doctor for a prescription. See the appendix "Keto-Green 16 Resources" on how to obtain this system for your own use.

Why 16?

When I developed this diet, I did not select the figure of sixteen days arbitrarily (although I love the idea of "sweet sixteen"!). I happened to know that in numerology, the number 16 symbolizes the energy required to make decisive goals and pursue them—which we certainly need to become the healthy, vibrant individuals we're meant to be. But from a scientific and medical standpoint, I knew that within just fourteen to sixteen days, we doctors can measure discernible and positive changes in a person's physiology, weight, body composition, and metabolism—changes that happen quite quickly when dietary shifts are made. We don't have to wait months and months.

Based on my 2019 studies and other clinical research, the following benefits can potentially be achieved in just sixteen days.

Drop Pounds Fast

In a study of thirty-eight obese patients conducted at the Charles University Medical Faculty in Prague in 1990, three groups were put on a high-protein, low-carbohydrate diet (similar to a ketogenic diet). The groups' diets varied in the number of calories, but were all low-calorie diets. After sixteen days, the average weight loss among participants was between eighteen and twenty-three pounds—over a pound a day! Though probably not typical for most dieters, that's pretty impressive and goes to show what the right mix of nutrients can do. Comparatively, in my own studies, participants lost up to a pound a day, on average.

Protect Your Cardiovascular Health

In 2003 Australian researchers studied eighteen women and thirteen men, ages twenty to seventy years old, to compare the effects of two lipid-lowering diets on risk factors for cardiovascular disease. One of the diets was similar to my Keto-Green diet because it was enriched with good fats—monounsaturated fatty acids, or MUFAs. The other diet was a high-carbohydrate/low-fat diet. Both diets were high in a phytochemical called lycopene, found in tomatoes, papaya, mangos, red cabbage, and red bell peppers (foods that are also on the Keto-Green 16 plan).

The participants followed one diet for fourteen to sixteen days, then switched over to the other diet for another fourteen to sixteen days. That way, each patient served as his or her own control. At the end of the study, the researchers concluded that the MUFA-enriched diet was the heart-healthier of the two. The MUFA diet significantly lowered triglycerides in the blood and raised HDL cholesterol (the "good" cholesterol, for which higher numbers are better). Both of these factors play a huge role in enhancing heart health. What's wonderful is that these changes happened in just sixteen days.

I was encouraged by this study, since heart disease is the leading killer of women, and it can be prevented by eating healthy fats and plant foods high in lycopene. Plus, this study shows that you can overturn cardiovascular risk factors in a relatively short time.

The results of my own studies also found a blood pressure advantage. Normal blood pressure is vital to heart health. When your blood pressure is taken, it's expressed in two numbers—one number on top (systolic) and one on the bottom (diastolic), like a fraction. For example, 120/75 mm Hg is ideal.

Systolic pressure refers to the amount of pressure in your arteries during the contraction of your heart muscle. Diastolic pressure measures your blood pressure when your heart muscle is between beats. Both numbers are important in determining your heart health. Numbers higher than ideal indicate that your heart is working too hard to pump blood throughout your body. Most participants in my studies were able to reduce their diastolic blood pressure by several points to reach 80 or below.

Get Control over Insulin and Glucose Rapidly

Keto-Green 16 is abundant in high-fiber vegetables, which help with glucose and insulin control and regulation of the hunger hormones. There is also a vegan version of the diet, which further amps up these veggies.

I included this plan for vegetarians and vegans, as well as anyone who wants to take a break from animal foods. Fasting from meat and other animal products is beneficial for your health—and a smart move to do at least once or twice a year for sixteen days each time.

Here's an example of what I'm talking about: After only sixteen days on a diet free of meat, dairy, and eggs (like my Vegan Keto-Green 16 plan), many people with type 2 diabetes might be able to get off insulin altogether, with a doctor's permission. This rather amazing outcome was shown in a study of a vegan-type diet high in plant fiber that was followed by twenty lean participants receiving insulin therapy for diabetes. They followed the diet for an average of sixteen days. Over the course of the study, doctors were able to lower the daily doses of insulin for each patient. Eleven patients discontinued insulin injections altogether. This study is a remarkable example of what can happen in just sixteen days, especially in terms of regulating insulin.

Alter Your Gut Bacteria for the Better

Inside your gut are trillions of healthy bacteria, collectively known as your microbiome. They work to metabolize nutrients, make vitamins, and detoxify harmful forms of estrogen that you are exposed to from the environment.

Scientists have found that people who live traditional, natural-food lifestyles (which population studies suggest are probably alkaline) have higher gut microbiota diversity than city dwellers. In one experiment, U.S. and Venezuelan researchers analyzed the microbiota of seven urban dwellers (five adults and two children), then had them stay in a rainforest village for sixteen days. When their samples were analyzed again, the results showed that their microbiota had changed to resemble the healthier condition of the local villagers.

Digestive health also improved in most of the participants in my studies. Participants reported less constipation, bloating, gas, spells of diarrhea, nausea, and heartburn.

This all goes to show that with natural foods such as vegetables and fruits, you can alter your gut flora for the better—and do it in as few as sixteen days.

Lose Inches Quickly

Candidates for weight-loss surgery are often put on low-calorie diets prior to surgery in order to further reduce their body fat. Usually these diets are of short duration, and they restrict fattening foods—similar to Keto-Green 16. The results can be quite remarkable. Researchers at the William Beaumont Army Medical Center in El Paso, Texas, for instance, put forty very obese people on a 1,000-calorie-a-day diet for fourteen days prior to weight-loss surgery. Thirty-eight patients lost weight on the diet, with an average loss of 5.2 pounds. Twenty-five patients lost three inches of fat around their waistlines—pretty impressive for just fourteen days of dieting.

In my studies, the loss of inches at the waistline was just as notable—between one and three inches on average.

So—are sixteen days meaningful and magical? You bet they are. A lot can happen in sixteen days. Isn't that sweet!

Part Two

Combine Keto and Alkaline
for Quick Weight Loss

Chapter 3

The 16 Keto-Green Foods

. . . .

What to eat for weight loss and good health is one of the most hotly debated topics around—even on ketogenic, alkaline diets. Eat this, don't eat that, and so goes the conflicting chatter about food. Fat is a good example. Based on old assumptions, we've long been told that eating fat will make us fat and that eating fat clogs our arteries. But now we know that none of this is clinically correct! Many scientific studies have made it clear that excess carbohydrates and sugars are the true causes of unhealthy weight and heart disease—and definitely not dietary fat, as previously suggested.

I can't imagine my life without Keto-Green fats such as fish, olive oil, avocados, and nuts. Eating a diet with good fats fuels you with energy, provides the building blocks of hormones, helps your body better absorb fat-soluble vitamins, sharpens your brain, and keeps you fuller for longer—with no cravings, just stronger willpower.

To cut down on any nutritional confusion on my Keto-Green plan, I've outlined exactly what to eat for weight loss, fat-burning, hormone balance, ketosis, alkalinity, and health. To make things even easier, I've narrowed the choices down to sixteen Keto-Green approved foods. No long shopping lists either!

A majority of these foods have special hormonal-balancing, fat-burning, and alkaline-forming properties. They regulate the speed at which your body burns fat, the power you have over weight-control hormones, and the types of bacteria in your gut. As you make these choices, your brain and body will reward you with rapid weight loss, a smaller waist, fewer cravings, and more energy.

Foods to Choose

Your lunches and dinners are planned around sixteen foods, which I'll talk about in the following sections.

Keto-Green Proteins

Fish (Salmon and White Fish)
Eating fish is always a good move for shedding pounds and inches. Fish is a terrific source of clean-burning protein. It helps keep you satisfied for longer, supports muscle development and repair, and boosts metabolism, making it great for keeping pounds at bay.

Salmon is often praised as one of the most nutritious foods in the world because it boasts endless health-boosting benefits. It is rich in nutrients, such as omega-3 fatty acids (known to promote heart and brain health) and iron, calcium, and selenium (minerals that support health and immunity).

I like salmon mostly for its omega-3 fats, which can cause body fat to melt away, especially around the waist. Scientists in Japan discovered that omega-3 fats in fish oil turn "bad" fat cells into healthy ones that incinerate calories like a furnace. The study focused on two types of body fat. There's the white kind, which turns the extra calories we eat into body fat stored in the belly, as a muffin top, and on our thighs. Then there are "beige" fat cells, that burn off calories—meaning they're metabolically active. These are the ones we all wish we had more of. Fish oil works by transforming white fat cells into beige ones. This benefit becomes especially important from middle age onward, when the number of "good" fat cells begins to decline and results in what we commonly call middle-age spread.

The omega-3s in salmon, as well as other seafood and shellfish like oysters (my favorite), help improve insulin sensitivity. This means insulin is working as it should and belly fat is less likely to form. Among other things, these fats help discourage the formation of agents that can trigger inflammation in the body, and they protect cell membranes from destruction by these agents. These fats also activate thyroid hormones for a faster metabolism.

Omega-3 fats replace excessive amounts of omega-6 and omega-9 fats (found in red meat) that are readily oxidized—factories for free radicals. In short, if you eat too much omega-6 and omega-9 fat, these fatty acids can overwhelm and dominate activity in cells, causing destruction. Eating more omega-3 fats can right this balance.

For variety, enjoy white fish too, such as cod, halibut, or flounder, which tend to be lower in toxins than other forms of seafood. The best thing about white fish is that it is a filling source of protein, selenium, and B vitamins, all vital for energy production, metabolism, immunity, and skin health. White fish is also thyroid-protective. Including it in your diet is a good strategy for burning away unwanted fat cells.

Please buy wild-caught fish whenever possible because it contains fewer environmental pollutants (which can interfere with the normal functioning of your hormones).

Chicken (White or Dark Meat)

Adding chicken to your diet is another good move. It's high in metabolism-stoking protein, important for boosting growth hormone, testosterone, and glucagon.

Protein requires the most calories to metabolize, with 20 to 30 percent of all the protein calories expended by your body to digest and absorb that nutrient, compared to fat and carbohydrates (zero to 3 percent for fat and 5 to 10 percent for carbs). So if you eat 100 calories' worth of protein, you effortlessly burn 20 to 30 calories of it.

You don't want to go overboard on protein or mistake a keto diet for a high-protein diet. If you consume more protein than your body requires, some of its amino acids will be converted into glucose via a process called gluconeogenesis. This becomes problematic and can kick you out of ketosis. We still need a mix of protein, fat, and alkalinizing foods to have a healthy fat-burning metabolism.

Please purchase organically raised, antibiotic-free, free-range chicken.

Beef (Grass-Fed)

I love beef and bison, but that's not why they're on my list. Beef helps create calorie-burning muscle, boosts the growth of brain cells, and combats sexual dysfunction. The protein it contains boosts growth hormone, testosterone, and glucagon. On my Keto-Green 16 diet, eating beef or bison supports ketosis, which leads to rapid weight loss as your fat stores are tapped into for energy.

Beef has few equals as a protein source, and it has an amino acid profile that's second to none. Besides the protein, B vitamins, carnitine, iron, zinc, and other nutrients, when beef is trimmed of excess visible fat and cooked appropriately, it delivers relatively low amounts of saturated fat.

Please purchase beef from free-range grass-fed cattle, or try free-range bison. Both contain higher concentrations of essential nutrients and omega-3 fatty acids, but no artificial hormones or contaminants. One of the biggest culprits in environmentally driven estrogen and progesterone imbalances are hormones in conventionally raised, non-grass-fed beef.

Keto-Green Alkalinizing Vegetables

Dark Leafy Greens (Raw or Cooked)

At the grocery store, my shopping cart can sometimes be mistaken for a lush green jungle. Some of my favorite green veggies are spinach, kale, beet greens, mustard greens, collard greens, arugula, Swiss chard, and lettuces of all varieties. I eat greens every single day, and I love them.

Dark leafy greens are the biggest celebrity of the Keto-Green 16 diet. They are highly alkalinizing to the body, and an alkaline body is healthier, with ample minerals, more calorie-burning muscle mass, and fewer toxins. Hormonally, an alkaline diet assists the body in burning fat, because (along with a low-carb diet) it decreases levels of belly-fat-forming cortisol.

What's more, just one serving a day of greens is beneficial to the brain. It helps prevent mental decline as a result of aging, according to a 2018 study published in *Neurology*.

Sprouts

People are always knocking sprouts. They say they don't taste good. They say they don't smell good. But I adore them and have been telling people for years to eat raw sprouts.

I promoted sprouts to my list of the top sixteen Keto-Green foods for two reasons. First, sprouts provide many nutrients, but their unique contribution is a group of compounds called glucosinolates (especially in broccoli sprouts). These natural chemicals support liver detoxification and help eliminate toxic, fat-forming, environmental estrogens from the body. Both actions clear the way for steady fat loss. Second, sprouts make your body more insulin sensitive, which means it's easier to turn the nutrients you eat into energy.

Choose from many different sprouts, including alfalfa, bean, broccoli, and radish. I particularly enjoy them in salads.

Cabbage

Cabbage, whether cooked or raw, is another detoxifying veggie, which is why it's on the list. Cabbage shifts excess, toxic estrogen out of your system. It's more difficult for your body to burn fat when toxins stand in the way.

Red cabbage, in particular, is a potent fat fighter. It contains phytonutrients called anthocyanins that have been shown to help reduce weight, particularly belly fat. (Also rich in anthocyanins are black soybeans, a food allowed on my Vegan Keto-Green 16 diet.)

A study published in the *Journal of Medicinal Food* reported that people who regularly consume anthocyanins lost 30 percent more belly fat over ninety days than a control group. It turns out that anthocyanins stimulate muscle cells to burn harmful visceral fat for energy. Other studies show that anthocyanins switch off chemical messengers that allow belly fat cells to absorb new fat.

Cabbage is a member of the cruciferous family of vegetables.

Other Cruciferous Vegetables

Many of us need to eat more cruciferous vegetables such as broccoli, cauliflower, Brussels sprouts, bok choy, and watercress. These veggies, both cooked and raw, contain indole-3 carbinol (I3C) and diindolylmethane (DIM), substances that detoxify harmful estrogen molecules and turn them into weaker, less cancer-promoting forms. Cruciferous veggies also release sulfur-containing nutrients that help the liver detoxify and block cancer cell formation. In short, these veggies support the body's natural detoxification system, help haul out metabolic trash, and leave our bodies free to burn fat.

Garlic and Other Alliums

You're probably familiar with garlic's flavor credentials, but how much do you know about its anti-obesity qualities? For one thing, garlic may help to regulate the formation of fat cells in our body by controlling inflammation, which underlies many diseases and makes your body resistant to losing weight. Through the activity of the inflammatory system, immature fat cells (pre-adipocytes) are converted into fat cells (adipocytes). Garlic contains anti-inflammatory compounds that may help inhibit this conversion by preventing the inflammation that turns immature fat cells into full-fledged fat cells. This helps prevent weight gain. Garlic can also increase adiponectin concentrations in the body.

Garlic is a member of the allium family, which also includes onions, leeks, scallions, and chives. All of these are rich sources of quercetin, a type of phytochemical that helps in activating enzymes essential for breaking down fats. Quercetin is an anti-inflammatory compound too. It suppresses the production of pro-inflammatory chemicals that stimulate growth of the fat tissues. Onions, in particular, are also loaded with chromium, which improves insulin sensitivity and reduces high blood sugar levels.

Keto-Green Fats

MCT Oil or Coconut Oil

I'm a big fan of medium-chain triglyceride oil, otherwise known as MCT oil, because so much research confirms that it is a bona fide fat burner. For example, a 2007 study of overweight, diabetic volunteers in China found that MCT oil effectively trimmed belly fat and overall body fat, compared to a control group who supplemented with corn oil only.

MCT oil is a special type of fat derived mainly from coconut oil. It is a beneficial oil to include while going Keto-Green because it is the easiest fat for the body to convert into ketones. In addition, MCT oil boosts metabolism and satiety, and it helps regulate blood sugar. MCT oil has been shown to increase the release of leptin and thus promote the feeling of fullness in the body.

Although MCT oil is made from coconut oil, they're not the same thing. Coconut oil contains four types of MCTs: C6, C8, C10, and C12. (The numbers refer to the length of the carbon chains.) Among these, the most superior is C8, caprylic acid, and you should look for an oil that consists mostly of C8 (around 5.5 grams per serving). It has the best ketone-producing and fat-burning profile. In fact, C8 is the MCT that's metabolized fastest, and it bypasses liver processing entirely and is therefore less likely to be stored as body fat.

Another benefit of C8 is that it helps support a healthy gut due to its powerful antimicrobial properties. It's able to eliminate harmful bacteria without interfering with good bacteria.

Coconut oil is permitted too. Although most cooking oils have a neutral pH, coconut oil is alkalinizing. According to a study published in *The Journal of Nutrition,* people who regularly eat coconut oil burn 65 percent more calories, even at rest.

Both MCT oil and coconut oil can be used for cooking, in salad dressings, drizzled over vegetables, or added to your morning coffee or tea, as in my Keto Coffee or Tea recipe (page 203). Adding one of these oils to your morning beverage staves off hunger too. I prefer MCT oil, however, because of its stronger fat-burning capability.

Olive Oil

Besides the alkalinity factor, there's one other main difference between conventional keto diets and my Keto-Green 16 diet: Mine plays up good fats such as olive oil, coconut oil, and other plant-based fats, as opposed to the full-fat dairy, cheeses, bacon, and fatty meats emphasized in most keto diets.

A big reason plant-based fats take center stage on the Keto-Green 16 plan is that they bust menopausal symptoms, such as weight gain, brain fog, mood swings, hot flashes, and fatigue, by helping to balance your hormones and keep you functioning at your best.

One of the best Keto-Green fats you can eat is olive oil. It has an impressive résumé of health perks, especially for women. For example, olive oil balances one of our major hormones, insulin. Recall that when our bodies have trouble using insulin and it stockpiles in the blood, we become insulin-resistant (the result of habitually eating a high-carb diet). Insulin resistance is one of the chief causes of belly fat. When scientists reporting in *Diabetes Care* looked at olive oil, they found those eating an olive-oil-rich diet had increased insulin sensitivity and lowered blood sugar after eating.

Olive oil can also help improve your body shape—less body fat and more toned curves. Researchers in Brazil studied forty-one adult women with excess body fat to see how extra-virgin olive oil affected their body composition (the relative amount of fat and muscle on one's frame). The control group ate a high-fat breakfast made with soybean oil; the other group ate one made with olive oil. No dietary changes were made other than the addition of these vegetable oils to their breakfasts.

After nine weeks, the olive oil group lost an average of five to six pounds, most of it fat tissue, whereas the control group lost two pounds on average. The researchers concluded, "Our results indicate that extra-virgin olive oil should be included into energy-restricted programs for obesity treatment." Their study was published in the *European Journal of Nutrition* in 2018.

The researchers did not say why olive oil had a fat-burning effect, but I suspect it is related to fighting inflammation and balancing hormones. A study published in the *International Journal of Food Sciences and Nutrition* in 2017 noted that an olive-oil-supplemented diet increases the fat-burning hormone adiponectin. Also, olive oil is one way to bring another hormone—testosterone—back up to healthy levels. This Keto-Green fat is a must for healthy hormones.

As for the best type of olive oil to purchase, I suggest a variety known as fresh-pressed extra-virgin olive oil. This means the manufacturer has put the olives into the crusher as fast as possible, within four hours of picking. The taste, purity, and health benefits of the oil are then preserved. So is the content of beneficial compounds called polyphenols found in olives.

For variety and to pump up fat intake, the Keto-Green 16 diet allows two other keto-friendly fats: butter and ghee. Ghee is purified butter that is void of milk proteins.

Nuts: Brazil Nuts, Almonds, Hazelnuts, and Pili Nuts

A food myth I need to crack is that nuts are fattening. Frankly, the opposite is true—as long as you eat nuts in small amounts. The Nurses' Health Study, which investigated approximately 51,000 healthy, middle-aged women for eight years, concluded that higher nut consumption was not associated with weight gain, and that it may even help control weight.

Here's why: The fiber in nuts works as a prebiotic, meaning that it feeds the good bacteria (probiotics) in our gut. Probiotics help in everything from aiding digestion to boosting metabolism and burning fat.

Also, nuts support weight control in another way: the fat, fiber, and protein they contain all work together to make us feel fuller and satiated longer. Nuts contain very few carbs, making them perfect for my Keto-Green 16 diet.

Various nuts are hormone-supportive too. In general, they amplify adiponectin in the body, prevent insulin resistance, and contain phytoestrogens, which may help guard against breast cancer. Phytoestrogens are natural compounds found in plant-based foods that affect you in the same way as estrogen produced by the body.

My top picks for nuts on this plan are almonds, Brazil nuts, hazelnuts, and pili nuts because they are the most alkaline-forming, compared to other nuts.

Avocado

Here's my must-have favorite fat for hormonal balance—the wonderfully delicious and versatile avocado. Avocados are truly a superfood, with studies showing benefits that range from fighting inflammation to improving insulin regulation and weight loss.

The majority of fat in an avocado is monounsaturated fat, which is very heart-healthy! An average avocado has about 22 grams of fat and almost 240 calories, keeping hunger at bay and insulin levels stable.

I love that insulin is managed well by the monounsaturated fats in avocados, while the fat also provides the building blocks the body needs to make both estrogen and progesterone. The fat in avocados lubricates the digestive system as well, and may in turn help to improve mild constipation.

Highly alkaline, avocados support weight control, as several clinical studies suggest. A study of twenty-six overweight adults, for example, suggested that one-half an avocado eaten at lunch significantly reduced hunger and desire to eat, and increased satiety as compared to a control meal that did not include an avocado. Additionally, several trials found that diets featuring avocados and other monounsaturated fats help fight belly fat and prevent diabetic health complications.

If you eat avocados regularly, congratulations—you may be

among a group of people who are very well nourished. Avocados are loaded with a lot of nutrients in which most people are deficient: dietary fiber, vitamins K and E, potassium, and magnesium.

Digestive and Alkaline-Support Foods

Sauerkraut, Kimchi, and Pickled Ginger

Sauerkraut is fermented cabbage, and kimchi is a Korean dish of fermented vegetables. Fermentation is the process by which yeast or bacteria convert sugar to alcohol; it creates conditions that promote the growth of beneficial probiotics, which are also found in products like yogurt and kefir. Research has shown fermented foods can support weight loss in at least a few ways.

In a study in *Nutrition Research,* participants ate unfermented kimchi vegetables for a month and then switched over to fermented kimchi for another month. After eating the fermented kimchi, they normalized their cholesterol and improved their carbohydrate metabolism. Plus they lost weight compared to when they ate the unfermented kimchi vegetables.

Both kimchi and sauerkraut are low in calories and high in fiber. High-fiber diets keep you fuller for longer, regulating leptin and ghrelin, and help you naturally reduce the number of calories you eat each day. Fiber also helps increase fat-burning, insulin-lowering adiponectin.

Their high probiotic content may also contribute to a trimmer waistline. The exact reasons aren't yet fully understood, but scientists believe that probiotics may have the ability to reduce the amount of fat your body absorbs from your diet. A study published in *Obesity* in 2017 found that supplementing with probiotics helped women lose belly fat—which is why I advocate eating probiotic foods and taking probiotic supplements.

Normally a garnish on a plate of sushi, pickled ginger is a true superfood. It has powerful anti-diabetic properties, meaning that it controls insulin and blood sugar. It also calms and supports the digestive system, fights inflammation, and is loaded with health-giving antioxidants. A small piece chewed before a meal helps get your digestive juices flowing, which maximizes the absorption of nutrients from food.

Pineapple, Mango, or Papaya

Fruit is nature's candy, right? So why wouldn't it be perfect on a weight-loss diet? True, many diets allow fruit for their fiber and nutrient content—but I've limited fruit on the Keto-Green 16 plan because most have high concentrations of sugar and will block fat-burning.

However, you may choose small amounts of three digestion-supporting fruits—pineapple, mango, and papaya. All three contain natural enzymes that help your body digest protein and carbohydrates. We need more enzymes as we get older, because our bodies produce less of them over time. These fruits are also excellent inflammation fighters.

Papaya and mango are alkaline-forming, while pineapple is slightly acidic.

Choose one small serving after dinner, if you wish, to soothe digestion overnight. But if you find that these fruits lower ketosis, do not eat them. As for alkalinity, switch to papaya or mango if eating pineapple makes your body too acidic.

Bone Broth

Bone broth is a simple stock made from animal or fish bones, cooked over many hours. The long cooking time breaks down the connective tissues, releasing important nutrients and minerals that make this an almost magical elixir of health. Studies have shown that the longer you cook the broth (more than eight hours is best), the more minerals are extracted from the bones.

Bone broth is incredibly healing, especially when sipped by itself, because all the nutrients are absorbed directly into your bloodstream rather than being used up in the process of digesting other food.

My clients tell me they just love bone broth. It is so alkalinizing and supportive of balanced hormones and overall health. It helps with digestion, joint function, immunity, and virtually every other function in the body. It's also high in magnesium, which most of us are deficient in, and calcium, important for strong bones. It also doesn't hurt that bone broth helps us release that stubborn, unhealthy weight.

One of my favorite benefits of bone broth is that it is a natural source of collagen. Boosting collagen has a number of health benefits and very few known risks. For starters, collagen improves skin health by reducing wrinkles and dryness—a benefit I see every time I drink a lot of bone broth. Collagen may also help increase muscle mass, prevent bone loss, and relieve joint pain.

A daily mug of bone broth is perfect to support this plan. It is soothing, enhances satiety, reduces caloric intake, helps in weight loss, and keeps you hydrated.

Bone broth prepared at home is your best option. Making it couldn't be easier: see my recipe on page 220. I also have a recipe for a vegan alkaline broth on page 221.

Lemons or Limes

Stock up on lemons or limes. You'll use their fresh juice to make my Alkalinizing Detox Beverage every morning. Outside the body, both are acidic fruits with a pH of 2, but they have great alkalinizing effects inside the body. Lemons and limes are rich in polyphenols—active plant compounds that have anti-obesity, anti-inflammatory, liver-detox, and insulin-controlling benefits.

THE SEXY, SLIM, AND YOUNGER 16 AT A GLANCE

1. Fish (salmon and white fish)
2. Chicken (light and dark meat)
3. Beef, grass-fed
4. Dark leafy greens, raw or cooked
5. Sprouts, raw
6. Cabbage, cooked or raw
7. Other cruciferous vegetables, cooked or raw
8. Garlic and other alliums

9. MCT oil or coconut oil
10. Olive oil
11. Nuts—Brazil nuts, almonds, hazelnuts, pili nuts
12. Avocado
13. Sauerkraut, kimchi, and pickled ginger
14. Pineapple, mango, and papaya
15. Bone broth
16. Lemons and limes

Serving Sizes of Keto-Green Foods

If you follow the sixteen-day meal plan to the letter, your daily serving sizes are automatically calculated for you. It's perfectly fine, however, to adjust your portion size upward if needed. A 200-pound man will have higher requirements (say, 6 ounces of protein and an extra cup of veggies at meals) than, for example, a woman who weighs 120 pounds (who might have 4 ounces of protein and smaller servings of vegetables at meals).

I give serving sizes as guidelines only. Check your fullness as a guide too. Eat only until you're satisfied but not stuffed. I love the rule followed by the healthy, long-living Okinawans: They recite a 2,500-year-old Confucian mantra before meals that reminds them to stop eating when their stomachs are 80 percent full.

If you plan some of your own meals around these sixteen foods, you'll want to measure your serving sizes. Many people can't quite picture what a moderate serving is, but they have a God-given food gauge—the palm of their hand. No matter what you eat, it should be able to fit inside the palm of your hand (not including your fingers!). The palm of your hand is considered a medium-sized (or moderate) portion.

On days when you opt to create do-it-yourself meals from the food list, plan your meals according to these flexible guidelines:

- Protein: 4 to 6 ounces, or a palm-sized serving at lunch and dinner

- Alkalinizing vegetables: 1 to 2 cups at lunch and dinner (can be combined, such as 1 cup greens + ¼ cup chopped onions + ¾ cup broccoli). Feel free to have more of these vegetables to assist with alkalinity.

- Fats: Have up to six servings daily, and choose from the following:

  MCT oil or coconut oil: 1 tablespoon = 1 fat serving
  Olive oil, ghee, or butter: 1 tablespoon = 1 fat serving
  Nuts: ½ cup = 1 fat serving
  Nut butter: 1 tablespoon = 1 fat serving
  Avocado: ½ avocado = 1 fat serving

  Fats are great at controlling hunger—so you can have an even larger fat allotment to assist with satiety, if needed.

- Sauerkraut or kimchi: ½ cup to 1 cup daily. Or pickled ginger, 4 to 5 slices daily

- Pineapple, mango, or papaya: Have 1 ring pineapple (1¼ inches thick) or ½ cup cubed mango or papaya daily after dinner.

- Lemon and lime juice (fresh is preferred): for your morning Alkalinizing Detox Beverage (page 74), and can be used liberally in oil-based salad dressing

- Bone broth: 1 to 2 cups daily or more if hungry (page 220)

OPTIONAL ADD-IN FOODS

- Unsweetened nut milks such as almond or coconut milk, coconut milk kefir, or coconut water kefir—limit to 1 cup daily. If you use store-bought brands, check the label for carbohydrate content in order to keep your carbs under 40 grams a day.

- Eggs. These can be used in cooking and can help curb hunger. My Egg Hand Salad recipe is a delicious way to eat eggs.

- Seasonings (with no added sugar) such as Himalayan sea salt, black pepper, dried parsley, lemon pepper, cumin, turmeric, paprika, chili powder, cayenne pepper, garlic powder, onion powder, and Italian seasoning.

- Vegetarian swaps: tempeh, miso, black soybeans, vegan protein powder, nuts, portabella mushrooms. See my sixteen-day Vegan Keto-Green 16 plan in Chapter 6 for how to follow a 100 percent plant-based diet.

Foods to Avoid

Perhaps you tried "going keto" in the past, but without the results you expected. It might have been because you weren't doing the keto part correctly. You might have been eating some very healthy foods, but they may have been keto-dirty and not keto-clean, as I discussed previously. These foods can upset your body chemistry, keeping you from attaining ketosis or booting you out of it.

The whole purpose of the Keto-Green diet is to help your body stay in ketosis and stay alkaline—without side effects like "keto flu," moodiness, or nutrient deficiencies—and help you feel sexy, lean, and beautiful. All of this happens when you root out certain foods that you assume are keto-friendly but are not. Remove these foods, replace them with delicious keto-friendly swaps, and wonderful things happen.

Here's a rundown of types of foods to avoid while following the Keto-Green 16 plan for the next sixteen days:

Dairy foods, including cheeses (although dairy is permitted on some keto diets, it can be a roadblock to healthy progress for many people)

Grains and cereals

Pastas

Flours, wheat, and any gluten-containing grain or product

Sugars and syrups

Any food with added sugar or carbohydrates

Artificial sweeteners

Artificially sweetened drinks, such as diet sodas

Candy, pastries, all sweets

Starchy vegetables such as potatoes, yams, sweet potatoes, root vegetables, peas, corn, popcorn, legumes, lentils, and so forth

Juices (except fresh lemon and lime juice)

Processed foods

Most fruits, except those on the food list

Cured meats and cold cuts (from meat that is not grass-fed)

Margarines and trans fats

Alcohol (but if you want a drink, limit yourself to one 5-ounce glass of low-sugar wine—preferably red—or 1½ ounces of tequila daily, though you should keep in mind that alcohol lowers inhibitions and thus reduces willpower to stick with a Keto-Green meal, and that you will achieve better results if you omit alcohol over the next sixteen days)

Understand which foods work with your body's fat-burning ability, not against it. When you go Keto-Green, you'll have peace of mind, knowing how to choose keto-friendly, alkaline-boosting, hormone-balancing foods that help you look better, feel better, and get glowing health.

This is a surefire sixteen-day plan that will boost your energy, clear your mind, and trim your waistline. Stick to it. You can do this—and lay a strong, healthy foundation for the rest of your life.

Chapter 4

The Fat-Loss Power
of Intermittent Fasting

. . . .

For many years, food dominated my thoughts. I was obsessed with what I was having for my next meal and the meal after that. All of this took up a lot of brain space. Then, while honing my Keto-Green formula, I discovered something called intermittent fasting. Among other things, it involved eating fewer meals (and fewer worries about what to eat).

This form of fasting started off as a way for me to lose pounds. As I designed my Keto-Green program I road-tested intermittent fasting myself regularly and found it to be quite cleansing physically, mentally, and emotionally. I had greater mental clarity and less angst about food. Best of all, intermittent fasting made it easier for me to lose weight and keep it off. It soon became a way of life. Nowadays I do it for its many other health benefits and just because it makes me feel so wonderful. I have more energy, greater inner calm, and sharper mental clarity. I no longer obsess about food, and I can't imagine intermittent fasting not being part of my routine for the rest of my life.

This form of fasting, also called "time-restricted feeding" in scientific jargon, is backed by solid research and has been garnering a lot of attention in diet circles. There are different types of intermittent fasting, but the type I recommend for this program involves sixteen hours of fasting. Don't worry: most of it takes place overnight, when you're sleeping. It's followed by an eight-hour window in which you eat lunch and dinner.

While not eating for sixteen hours may sound incredibly difficult to achieve, I bet you've already done some intermittent fasts. If you've had dinner, then slept late and not eaten again until lunch the next day, then you have practiced intermittent fasting.

If you really think about it from an evolutionary perspective, fasting has always been a part of our lives. Our bodies were programmed long ago to withstand periods of fasting when people depended on the natural cycles of day and night, with food primarily eaten during the day and fasting occurring at night. Fasting is our legacy and honors our evolutionary design!

Medically and metabolically, I learned through my research that intermittent fasting helps trigger ketosis, burn belly fat, restore hormonal balance, and assist the body in the elimination of toxins. With those benefits, it was the perfect complement to my Keto-Green 16 diet, so I integrated it into the plan.

I don't recommend jumping right into a sixteen-hour fast, however, but rather working up through twelve-, thirteen-, fourteen-, and fifteen-hour fasts. I'll show you how to do that in this chapter.

Intermittent Fasting: Your Weight and Your Waistline

I have lots of good news for you here, as intermittent fasting has a lot of benefits.

- **Maintains metabolism.** As a quick refresher, metabolism relates to how your body produces energy from food and how it stores that energy. Restricting calories (like most diets emphasize) can cause a metabolic logjam, in which the body burns fewer calories a day. However, a study published in the *British Journal of Nutrition* showed that fasting for short periods of time actually increases your metabolism—which means your body burns fat and calories faster.

- **Is a more effective weight-loss strategy than conventional calorie-cutting diets.** Studies have directly compared calorie restriction to intermittent fasting to see which strategy works best for fat loss. In a 2016 study published in the journal *Obesity*, researchers compared zero-calorie alternate-day fasting (a form of intermittent fasting) with daily caloric restriction in obese adults.

    What were the findings? Fat loss in the upper body, which includes the more dangerous fat packed in around the organs, was almost twice as high with fasting as opposed to calorie cutting. As for body fat, there was almost six times the amount of fat loss using fasting. Intermittent fasting helps you use up stored fat very effectively, especially when it's paired with keto-alkaline nutrition.

- **Burns belly fat.** Intermittent fasting is one of the best strategies you can use for fighting belly fat—for three reasons. First, intermittent fasting inhibits what's called alpha fat receptors. These are proteins in fat tissue that decrease fat-burning and restrict the amount of blood flow that passes through cells in the abdomen (we need good circulation to help burn fat). Having active alpha-2 receptors makes it difficult to get rid of belly fat.

    Second, your abdominal tissue has about 400 percent more receptors for the stress hormone cortisol, which makes it easier for the body to store fat in response to stress, than tissue elsewhere in the body. So intermittent fasting is not only good for your stress response but also good for preventing a certain degree of fat storage in response to stress.

    Third, intermittent fasting forces your body to get energy by converting tough-to-budge fat (including belly fat) into ketones and finding energy reserves beyond stored glucose (thus burning fat). This is one reason you'll often feel more energetic with this type of fasting.

A 2014 study found that people also lost 4 to 7 percent of their waist circumference with intermittent fasting. This indicates a significant loss of that harmful belly fat that builds up around your organs and causes disease.

- **Keeps fat off for good.** The vast majority of people who lose weight with a typical calorie-cutting diet will gain it back, and roughly two-thirds of them put on more pounds than they lost. This problem—called yo-yo dieting or rebound weight gain—can be prevented with intermittent fasting.

  Here's why. If you're overweight, by consistently reducing the amount of food you eat by 25–50 percent you will lose pounds and fat. This is called continuous calorie reduction, because you are continuously reducing what you eat—at every meal and snack, every day.

  Intermittent fasting *isn't* continuous calorie reduction per se, but rather an intermittent reduction, in which you're eating at specific times within a certain window. And you may not be cutting calories during that window.

  A lot of research strongly backs what I said earlier: it's hard to sustain a continuous calorie-reduced diet for a long time. This is why people gain so much weight after going off these diets. With intermittent fasting, you get similar weight and fat loss results, plus it's easier to stick with. That's why you're less likely to regain the pounds you've lost.

  Also, a big problem with continuous calorie reduction is that it forces the metabolism to slow down to the lowered calorie intake. If you return to eating a higher amount of calories after the diet, your now-slower metabolism makes weight regain inevitable. Intermittent fasting does the opposite—it increases your metabolism. I therefore recommend intermittent fasting as part of an overall strategy for staying slim after you've achieved your ideal weight.

- **Preserves calorie-burning muscle tissue.** Intermittent fasting gets criticized because some people believe that going without food, even for just sixteen hours, can cannibalize precious muscle. The opposite is true. One study showed that intermittent fasting causes less muscle loss than the more standard method of continuous calorie restriction. In fact, it showed that intermittent fasting is four times better at preserving lean mass.

- **Resolves insulin resistance.** Much research has found that intermittent fasting helps prevent insulin resistance (which, as you know by now, is responsible for weight gain and the most common cause of type 2 diabetes). A study reported in *Translational Research* showed that blood sugar dropped by 3–6 percent and fasting insulin levels were reduced by 20–31 percent. Further, a study published in the *World Journal of Diabetes* found that intermittent fasting in type 2 diabetics improved participants' body weight and glucose levels.

- **Clears away defective cells.** Intermittent fasting kick-starts autophagy. This is a process by which the body gets rid of cells that have a greater risk of becoming infected or cancerous. These are cells that also lead to accelerated aging, Alzheimer's disease, and type 2 diabetes. Think of autophagy like spring-cleaning—it tosses out the junk and clears the way for health and vitality.

    Eating, however, prevents autophagy. Even a little food triggers an enzyme called mTOR, a powerful inhibitor of autophagy. Too much mTOR can lead to obesity, diabetes, and neurodegenerative diseases. Low levels of mTOR have been found to decrease cancer risk, decrease inflammation, and improve insulin sensitivity, and may also increase longevity. This is why intermittent fasting supports good health.

- **Improves your gut and circadian rhythm.** Those trillions of healthy bacteria in the gut (the microbiome) are affected not only by what we eat but also by when we eat. In a study published in the scientific journal *Cell Metabolism*, researchers discovered that gut bacteria have their own circadian rhythm, like humans have—a clock of sorts, in which our physiological processes are synced to the twenty-four-hour solar cycle of light and dark. For example, your body starts to wind down and prepare for sleep after sunset, and it's programmed to wake up at sunrise.

When the microbiome's circadian rhythm is thrown off, there's trouble: brain fog, slower metabolism, insulin resistance, inability to burn fat, and impaired detoxification. What disrupts the microbiome's rhythm? Erratic eating patterns, eating all day, and night eating. Fortunately, intermittent fasting restores normal gut circadian rhythms and prevents these complications, allowing your digestive tract to rest and digest. This can also help to heal any damage that you may have done to your gut lining over the years.

The Hormonal Benefits of Intermittent Fasting

Here's where intermittent fasting really shines: balancing your weight-control hormones. When you fast, your body adjusts certain hormone levels to make stored body fat more accessible. Many of the hormones I discussed in Chapter 1 are affected positively by intermittent fasting, making it a powerful tool for fixing out-of-balance hormones. Here are specific changes that occur in hormones when you fast.

Estrogen

Estrogen is metabolized by your liver. This organ converts excess estrogen into breakdown products that can be eliminated from the body. Within the liver there are three main pathways through which estrogen can be metabolized. Only one is a healthy, happy choice. The other two can lead to cardiovascular issues and cancer. Your body will store estrogen in target tissues—in women, primarily the breasts. If estrogen goes down the wrong pathway, this can result in a significantly elevated risk of breast cancer.

Intermittent fasting helps prevent this from happening. It detoxes unhealthy estrogens and helps eliminate them from the body through the correct pathway.

Of utmost importance to women: In one study, breast cancer survivors who typically didn't eat for at least twelve and a half hours overnight had a 36-percent reduction in the risk of their breast cancer returning, compared with those who had shorter overnight fasts!

Also, if you're currently overweight and carrying a lot of body fat, your body may be producing too much estrogen for you, no matter what your age. Excess fat on your body is a mini-factory of estrogen since each fat molecule secretes its own estrogen for maintenance. Too much estrogen (a condition called estrogen dominance) can be fat-forming. Intermittent fasting helps lower your body fat; when that happens, estrogen drops to more normal and balanced levels.

As I explained earlier, intermittent fasting is good for your gut, and a healthy gut promotes healthy estrogen metabolism (which, along with weight control, is critical for reducing the risk of breast cancer).

Insulin and Glucagon

Intermittent fasting controls insulin and reduces insulin resistance. Research shows that it can lower blood sugar by 3 to 6 percent and reduce fasting insulin levels by 20 to 31 percent, thus helping protect against type 2 diabetes. In fact, intermittent fasting is one of the main tools I've used over the years to combat blood sugar issues and correct insulin problems in patients and clients.

When your body fasts and insulin drops, glucagon is released, causing the body to utilize alternative energy sources (such as fat stores) in the absence of glucose. Research shows that this hormone rises two-fold on the third day of intermittent fasting. This means it gets right to work unlocking fat stores!

Adiponectin and Growth Hormone

Intermittent fasting increases levels of adiponectin secreted by fat cells, as seen in studies of Ramadan fasting, which involves prolonged fasting for up to twelve hours during Islam's holy month of Ramadan.

As your body shifts to burning fat as its main source of energy during fasting, levels of adiponectin and growth hormone go skyward. Growth hormone can increase as much as five-fold. Both hormones go up for the sole purpose of mobilizing fat to provide energy and thus are responsible for a great deal of fat loss.

Because both of these hormones decrease as we age, leading to muscle loss and a slower metabolism, increasing them and bolstering their function is key to healthy living.

Cortisol

Recall that your abdominal tissue has about 400 percent more cortisol receptors than tissue in other parts of the body. This makes it easier for your body to store belly fat in response to stress. Intermittent fasting actually reduces the number of active cortisol receptors, so less fat gets stored around your midsection.

Leptin and Ghrelin

Intermittent fasting also plays an important role in regulating our hunger hormones. For example, leptin resistance, when the brain doesn't get the message to stop eating, is reduced with intermittent fasting. Your body becomes more leptin sensitive and thus can process hunger signals more efficiently, lowering your risk of overweight and obesity.

If you think you'll get too hungry by fasting, think again. Intermittent fasting has been shown to positively affect the hunger hormone ghrelin—with some super-beneficial results. Here's why. Maybe you wake up hungry—so you eat breakfast. A few hours later comes lunch. You might snack in between. Then it's dinner and time to eat again. Maybe you feel like snacking again just before going to bed.

The problem is that by eating every few hours, you're repeatedly hiking up your glucose levels. Along comes more and more insulin, and then you store fat. With every meal, this cycle repeats itself daily, making it very tough to lose weight because your body is always storing fat versus burning it.

With intermittent fasting, you wake up maybe a little hungry, but you don't eat. Yes, your ghrelin levels rise, but lots of positive things happen:

- Higher levels of circulating ghrelin correspond with an increased release of growth hormone by the pituitary gland. Remember, growth hormone is responsible for increased fat loss and muscle gain, and it's touted as an anti-aging hormone.

- Ghrelin supports dopamine production. Dopamine is the brain's natural feel-good chemical, producing emotions of happiness and satisfaction. Increased dopamine is why so many people say they feel great while fasting.

- Ghrelin is involved in protecting brain cells. It plays one of its biggest roles in the hippocampus, which is responsible for long- and short-term memory. Secreted in the stomach, this hormone can actually help you retain more memories. This is one of the reasons people say they have less brain fog and more mental clarity while fasting.

All of these hormonal benefits create the perfect conditions for burning fat more efficiently (especially belly fat), feeling energetic, and achieving mental clarity. What could be better?

OTHER MEDICAL ADVANTAGES OF INTERMITTENT FASTING

Medical studies have shown that intermittent fasting:

- Increases energy

- Improves cognition, memory, and clear thinking

- May improve immunity, lower diabetes risk, and improve heart health

- Slows down the growth of tumors and decreases cancer risk

- Reduces chronic inflammation (the underlying cause of many diseases in the body)

- Manages the symptoms of polycystic ovary syndrome (PCOS)

- Improves joint and bone health

- Protects the heart

- Reduces the risk of menstrual problems

- Improves mental health during the transition to menopause

- Improves mood

- Reduces symptoms and anxiety, stress, and depression, especially as related to obsessive thoughts over food and eating

Intermittent Fasting and Keto-Green 16: Guidelines

After I've enumerated all the benefits, I trust you're ready to put intermittent fasting into action. If so, how do you begin? Here are the guidelines.

- The ideal fasting window for this program is sixteen hours without food, skipping breakfast and restricting your eating period to eight hours, such as between 10 A.M. and 6 P.M. (which is what I do) or between 11 A.M. and 7 P.M. This is referred to as the 16/8 protocol. Thus, you'd finish your dinner by 6 or 7 P.M. each evening and not eat anything after dinner, except for *Keto Bone Broth* (page 220) or some herbal tea.

    Note: I recognize that many times it's difficult to finish eating by 7 P.M., but it is metabolically beneficial to do so. The later we eat, the more insulin is secreted; this can contribute to insulin resistance, which in turn creates greater fat stores.

- Upon awakening, follow this routine every morning:

    - Test your urinary pH and ketones first thing in the morning (and periodically throughout the day whenever you go to the bathroom), with the goal of keeping your pH at or above 7.0 and getting into moderate ketosis (pink on the test strip).

    - Prepare and drink either my Alkalinizing Detox Beverage or my Dr. Anna Cabeca Mighty Maca Plus drink. To make the Alkalinizing Detox Beverage: To a large glass of warm water, add ½ teaspoon lemon juice and ½ to 1 tablespoon unfiltered apple cider vinegar; if you're not alkaline, add ¼ to ½ teaspoon baking soda. To make the Mighty Maca Plus drink: To a large glass of warm water, add two scoops Mighty Maca Plus. When you're fasting, be doubly sure that you are taking in the healthiest nutrients that your body needs, nourishing your body at the cellular level. I find that my Mighty Maca Plus is one of the best ways to obtain extra nutrition and get alkaline. Aside from the hormone-balancing herb maca, Mighty Maca Plus also contains more than thirty other super-foods, including turmeric, which has been found to help prevent weight gain.

- Follow the Alkalinizing Detox Beverage or Mighty Maca Plus drink with a cup of coffee or herbal tea (such as cinnamon, chamomile, chai, or green tea with a cinnamon stick). Blend in 1 teaspoon to 1 table-spoon MCT oil or coconut oil to increase your fat in-take to boost ketosis. Do you like creamy coffee or tea? If so, add 1 teaspoon ghee, or coconut ghee if you're vegan. It mimics the creaminess that you get with milk or cream. I call this Keto Coffee or Tea. Both also stave off hunger and cravings.

   If you aren't getting the results you want, if you get hungry a lot, or if you have been diagnosed with diabetes or blood sugar problems, you may want to forgo coffee because it can raise cortisol and blood glucose and can kick you out of ketosis. Try an herbal tea instead.

- Eat your lunch (or brunch) sixteen hours after you finished dinner the night before—usually at 10 or 11 A.M.

- Have dinner, finishing by 6 or 7 P.M.

- Do not eat between meals. That advice might seem to fly in the face of conventional wisdom, but here's the truth: if you're over forty, snacking can be destructive to your goals. It can cause insulin resistance, weight gain, hot flashes, and inflammation. If you feel hunger pangs during the day, add more healthy fats, oils, and nuts to your meals. You can also increase your portion sizes. Another strategy is to drink some *Keto Bone Broth* (page 220) or a Dr. Anna Cabeca's

Keto-Alkaline Protein Shake midday, if needed. The hunger pangs will disappear, and you won't have to rely on will-power. This all gets easier. Eventually you'll retrain your body to not desire snacks, I promise.

Of course, you must remain focused on this nourishing diet when in your feeding window—you certainly can't eat donuts and drink sugary soda or sweet tea all day long and still expect to gain benefits from your Keto-Green 16 intermittent fast!

Levels of Intermittent Fasting

Not everyone can jump right into a 16/8 intermittent fasting proto-col schedule, however, which is why I have devised three categories of fasters—beginner, intermediate, and expert, each with a different fasting window.

Beginner

You are a beginner if:

- You have never tried intermittent fasting before.

- You are in the habit of eating breakfast as soon as you get up.

- You tend to feel hungry upon waking up.

- You know you have a lot of toxins stored up in your body because of the sluggish way you feel.

Recommendation: Ease into the practice. Fast overnight for only a twelve- to thirteen-hour window. If you finish dinner at 7 P.M., for example, follow the morning routine after you get up, then break your fast between 7 and 8 A.M. with one of my Keto-Green smoothies, made with the Keto-Green Meal Replacement or similar product (pages 204–217). Have an extra Keto-Green smoothie during your feeding window, and/or a cup of bone broth (page 220), or ¼ cup nuts. Go on to lunch and dinner; be sure to include a green salad.

Intermediate

You are an intermediate if:

- You have tried intermittent fasting a few times but have not followed a structured intermittent fasting plan.
- You sometimes skip breakfast.
- You normally don't feel hungry in the morning.

Recommendation: Shoot for a fourteen- to fifteen-hour fasting window overnight. If you finish dinner at 7 P.M., for example, follow the morning routine when you get up. Then plan to break your fast at 9 or 10 A.M. with a Keto-Green smoothie. If you feel hungry during your feeding window, have another Keto-Green smoothie, made with my Keto-Green Meal Replacement or similar product (pages 204–217), and/or a cup of *Keto Bone Broth* (page 220), or a Keto-Green salad.

Expert

You are an expert if:

- You routinely do intermittent fasting, particularly the 16/8 method.
- Intermittent fasting has become a habit, and you do not feel hungry in the morning, nor do you miss having breakfast.

Recommendation: Follow the 16/8 method exactly.

As a beginner or intermediate, you may become accustomed to intermittent fasting within several days. If so, feel free to "graduate" to expert and follow the 16/8 method.

That's really all there is to it. You'll find that intermittent fasting is easy to implement. You fast sixteen hours, half of which is overnight while sleeping. It's a type of *healthy* fasting that you can stick to and even embrace, especially if you're nourishing your body the Keto-Green way.

Optional Water Fasting: Days 14 to 16

Here's a way to supercharge your results and benefits: Do an optional water fast on the final two to three days of my plan. Water fasting is a type of fast that restricts everything except water, non-caffeinated herbal teas, and bone broth. As for water, drink at least 8 to 12 cups, spread out through the day.

Water fasting has health benefits, including weight loss and the stimulation of autophagy, the process that helps your body break down and recycle old parts of your cells.

If you are a beginner, consider doing a one-day water fast on day 16; if you're an intermediate, try water fasting on days 15 and 16; if you're an expert, do a water fast on days 14, 15, and 16.

When you break your fast on day 17, do so with a Keto-Green smoothie. Then resume the plan for another sixteen days, especially if you want to lose more weight and obtain great results.

Water fasting is completely optional. There are also some people who should *not* fast: people with diabetes, cancer, or any active disease, or if you're pregnant or lactating. If you think these forms of fasting may be right for you, be sure to consult your healthcare provider before getting started.

Chapter 5

The Breakthrough
Keto-Green 16 Diet Plan

. . . .

The next sixteen days will signal a new way of eating and a new way of life for you!

You'll immediately begin losing fat and inches. You'll eliminate hunger and cravings. You'll boost your metabolism, allowing your body to efficiently burn fat for energy. You'll experience laser-sharp thinking and focus. You'll stabilize your blood sugar and become more insulin sensitive, so you don't have to worry as much about high blood sugar, weight gain, and various menopausal symptoms — especially hot flashes (one cause of which is insulin resistance). You'll naturally detoxify your body from pollutants, chemicals, and hormone disruptors that keep you from losing weight. You'll prime yourself to make this a lifetime diet after the initial and amazing sixteen days are over.

All of this is possible because of the keto-alkaline forces at work in this diet. It is the perfect plan for fat loss and optimal health. Keto-Green eating naturally manages your body's weight-control hormones and keeps your body in a fat-loss environment.

Day by day, you'll see the number on your scale go down, which is exciting! By the end of sixteen days, you'll be significantly lighter, with pounds and inches gone like magic.

What follows is the exact Keto-Green 16 protocol: the basic actions you'll take daily, my meal planning guidelines, and suggested menus for the entire sixteen days.

Your Morning Routine

1. Test your urinary pH and ketones first thing in the morning (and periodically throughout the day whenever you go to the bathroom), with the goal of keeping your pH at or above 7.0. The greener the strip, the more alkaline your body. As for ketones, the pinker the strip, the higher your level of ketosis.

2. Upon rising, prepare and drink my Alkalinizing Detox Beverage: a large glass of warm water to which you've added ½ teaspoon lemon juice, ½ to 1 tablespoon unfiltered apple cider vinegar, and, if you're not alkaline, ¼ to ½ teaspoon baking soda. *Or* drink a large glass of warm water to which you've added two scoops Mighty Maca Plus (available on my website).

3. Follow the Alkalinizing Detox Beverage or Mighty Maca Plus drink with a cup of coffee or herbal tea (such as cinnamon, chamomile, chai, or green tea with a cinnamon stick). Add 1 teaspoon to 1 tablespoon MCT oil or coconut oil to increase your fat intake in order to boost ketosis. As I suggested earlier, if you like creamy coffee or tea, add 1 teaspoon ghee, or coconut ghee for vegans, and blend. It mimics the creaminess that you get with milk or cream. I call this Keto Coffee or Keto Tea. Both stave off hunger and cravings.

    It's worth repeating: if you aren't getting the results you want, if you feel hungry a lot, or if you have been diagnosed with diabetes or blood sugar problems, you may want to forgo coffee because it can raise cortisol and blood glucose and can kick you out of ketosis. Try an herbal tea instead.

4. Continue this morning routine each day for sixteen days.

Flexible Meal Planning

In working with thousands of women and men on this diet, one thing became clear: People like a certain amount of flexibility. Some people feel comfortable following a menu plan to the letter, while others like to pick and choose from the sixteen foods to plan their meals. Still others like to do a little of both.

If you prefer to devise your own Keto-Green 16 plan, all you need to do is follow the meal planning principles described in this chapter. They show you the basic structure of your lunches and dinners. Then use the list of sixteen foods on pages 59–60 as a guide for what to eat.

If you'd rather follow a menu plan with recipes to the letter—without having to think—simply follow the sixteen-day meal plan that begins on page 89. It gives you daily lunches and dinners that are delicious, satisfying, and guaranteed to take off inches and pounds.

Maybe you're somewhere in between—you like to try new recipes but also enjoy the independence of planning your own meals. It's fine to do both. Further, it's also okay to enjoy the same lunches and dinners a few days in a row if you have favorites.

Don't Forget Intermittent Fasting

It's a good idea to review the guidelines for intermittent fasting in Chapter 4, since it is so important to your success. Remember, you'll finish your dinner by 6 or 7 P.M. each evening, with no food or fluids overnight, with the exception of some herbal tea, water, or *Keto Bone Broth*, page 220 (vegans and vegetarians can do my *Keto Alkaline Broth*, page 221).

You'll eat your first meal of the day sixteen hours after you finished dinner the previous night, usually at 10 or 11 A.M. If you're a beginner or intermediate faster, you'll have a shorter fasting window—twelve to thirteen hours for beginners and fourteen to fifteen hours for intermediates—and you can break your fast earlier in the morning with a Keto-Green smoothie.

Building Your Meals

Remember, you can create your own meals, follow the menu plan exactly, or do a little of both. Here's a simple template for creating your meals.

Upon Awakening

Prepare and drink my Alkalinizing Detox Beverage or Mighty Maca Plus drink, followed by coffee or tea with 1 teaspoon to 1 tablespoon MCT oil, and optional 1 teaspoon coconut or regular ghee.

Lunch (11 A.M.)

Lunch = 1 protein serving + 1 to 2 servings alkalinizing vegetables + 1 to 2 fat servings

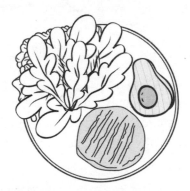

Examples:

- 1 pan-fried ground beef patty + 1 to 2 cups spinach, kale, or beet greens sautéed in 1 tablespoon olive oil or coconut oil + ½ avocado, sliced

- 1 serving cooked chilled salmon atop a bed of fresh greens, chopped raw cauliflower, and chopped onions; sprinkle with 1 tablespoon chopped almonds and toss with 1 tablespoon olive oil and lemon juice.

- Any of the lunch recipes provided

Dinner (finishing by 6 to 7 P.M.)

Dinner = 1 protein serving + 2 servings alkalinizing vegetables + 1 to 2 fat servings + digestive support food

After dinner, take two digestive enzyme supplements (see pages 126–127).

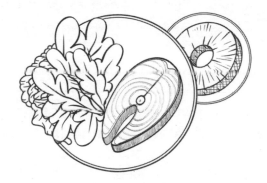

Examples:

- Baked chicken thigh + mashed cauliflower + side salad with fresh greens and 1 tablespoon chopped nuts tossed with 1 tablespoon olive oil and lemon juice + 1 serving of sauerkraut

- Steamed white fish atop 1 to 2 cups spinach, kale, or beet greens sautéed in 1 tablespoon olive oil or coconut oil, followed by ½ cup cubed mango or papaya or 1 ring pineapple

- Any of the dinner recipes provided

Snacking options

Although I do not recommend snacking, some people need Keto-Green snacks to curb hunger and cravings. If this describes you, feel free to include these snacks from the list of sixteen foods during your eight-hour feeding period:

- ¼ cup nuts

- ½ avocado drizzled with olive oil and sea salt

- Keto-Green shake or smoothie (see pages 204–218)

- 1 cup *Keto Bone Broth* (see page 220) or *Keto Alkaline Broth* (see page 221)

- 1 cup raw cruciferous veggies such as broccoli or cauliflower

- Hard-boiled egg

The Keto-Green Meal Replacement Option

You may replace any lunch or dinner with a Keto-Green shake or smoothie (pages 204–218), made with the Keto-Green Meal Replacement powder.

Also, have one of these smoothies whenever you feel you need a little extra fuel. If you're someone who deals with late-night food cravings, drink my Pineapple Keto-Green Smoothie (page 206) at 5 P.M. The fat and fiber it contains will fill you up.

Achieving Ketosis and Alkalinity

Within about four days, you should achieve ketosis. That's generally how long it takes to reach this fat-burning state, provided you're keeping your carbs at 40 grams or below daily, eating enough healthy fat, avoiding keto-dirty foods, and staying hydrated.

As for alkalinity, some people have trouble becoming alkaline, at least initially. To boost your body's alkalinity, try these hacks:

- Add ¼ to ½ teaspoon baking soda to your Alkalinizing Detox Beverage every morning.

- Briefly cook or sauté your greens to help your body fully absorb their nutrients.

- Double the green veggies in your salad, and add sprouts to your Keto-Green Meal Replacement smoothie.

- Add a chelated mineral supplement to your supplement regimen. Take magnesium at bedtime.

- Slow down your eating and chew your foods more thoroughly.

- Drink extra *Keto Bone Broth* (page 220) (or *Keto Alkaline Broth,* page 221—an option for vegans and vegetarians that is made with alkalinizing vegetables only).

- Make sure you're hydrating your body properly with enough filtered water in between meals.

- Drink 1 teaspoon to 1 tablespoon apple cider vinegar before your meals to help digestion and alkalinity.

- Use MCT oil or extra-virgin olive oil as the oil base in your salad dressings.

- Constipation contributes to acidity, so add a probiotic, magnesium supplement, vitamin C, and a fiber supplement until you are having daily bowel movements. You can also increase MCT oil or add cod liver oil at 1 tablespoon twice daily.

- Always purchase quality foods. Especially when it comes to fat, buying free-range, grass-fed, non-genetically-modified (non-GMO) foods becomes crucial. Whenever possible, choose organic, since conventional foods often grow in mineral-depleted, toxin-loaded soil.

- Look beyond the diet. Quality sleep is crucial to staying alkaline. So do stress management, exercise, and healthy bowel movements. Oxytocin, that wonderful hormone released when you hug, love someone, or have an orgasm, also creates alkalinizing benefits, so healthy relationships will help you stay alkaline too.

- And have fun!

HOW MUCH WATER SHOULD I DRINK?

Water is crucial to almost every function in the body. Without it, we can't absorb nutrients or eliminate toxins. It energizes you because water is used to make energy on a cellular level in your body. If you're even mildly dehydrated, your body will alert you with fatigue, and you'll feel wiped out. The more water, the better. My rule of thumb is to drink 60 to 70 ounces of pure water daily (not with meals, to avoid diluting important digestive enzymes). Use common sense, though—if you're a marathoner competing in the heat this summer, you need more, and if you're a sedentary worker indoors, you probably need less.

Be sure to *drink from the right container.* It was once customary to carry around a plastic water bottle as if it were a permanent extension of our arm. But now we know that plastic bottles contain the hormone disruptor and breast-cancer-linked substance bisphenol-A (BPA) and should be avoided.

But BPA-free plastic containers may be just as harmful. Animal studies have found that bisphenol-S (BPS), a replacement compound for BPA, may disrupt a cell's normal functioning, which could potentially lead to diabetes, obesity, asthma, birth defects, or even cancer.

So forget plastic water bottles. Always drink your water from a glass container or a stainless steel container (stainless steel is safest while you're driving).

Also, know what's in the water you drink and where it

comes from. Drinking water comes from a variety of sources, including public water systems and private wells. All sources of drinking water may contain contaminants. According to the Environmental Protection Agency and the Centers for Disease Control and Prevention, those contaminants include:

- Organic material suspended in the water of lakes, rivers, and streams from soil erosion

- Chemicals including nitrogen, bleach, salts, pesticides, heavy metals, toxins produced by bacteria, hormones, and human or animal drugs

- Biological contaminants such as bacteria, viruses, and parasites

- Radioactive contaminants like cesium, plutonium, and uranium

- Sewage releases

- Fertilizers and pesticides from farms and lawns

The presence of contaminants in water can lead to nasty health problems, including gastrointestinal illnesses, hormone disruption, reproductive problems, and neurological disorders. You may have heard about the catastrophic contamination of the water supply in Flint, Michigan, which had increased levels of lead in the drinking water. This was a result of improper water treatment and water pipe corrosion, which caused high levels of lead in children. High lead is known to increase mental illness, ADD, irrational behavior, and anger. Not coincidentally, Flint has been one of the most violent cities in the United States. Certainly the water supply played a role in this.

I know this all sounds scary, but you can easily avoid contaminated drinking water by purchasing a water filter. But what kind? Pitcher? Under the sink? Carbon block? Whole house? If you're not sure, the best course of action is to get a solid carbon block filter certified to NSF/ANSI 42, 53 and 401 (and NSF/ANSI 58, if you would like to add reverse osmosis). Reverse osmosis uses a partially permeable membrane to remove ions, molecules, and larger particles from drinking water.

Research suggests that alkaline water is the best liquid to drink, along with following an alkaline diet. Rich in alkalinizing minerals such as potassium, magnesium, calcium, and sodium, alkaline water offers many benefits: better hydration, rejuvenation, restoration and balance of pH, detoxification, and antioxidant support.

A 2016 study published in *Alternative Therapies in Health and Medicine* revealed that people who drink alkaline water have shown a lower incidence of heart disease, cancer, and total mortality. Alkaline water may also prevent osteoporosis and protect insulin-making cells in the pancreas.

It's easy to make alkaline water right at home. Simply add ½ teaspoon lemon juice (which makes water tastier), ½ to 1 tablespoon unfiltered apple cider vinegar, a pinch of cayenne pepper, and ½ teaspoon baking soda. Drink this right after waking up in the morning. There is also a wide range of water filters that can alkalinize your water. Mine is from Vollara.com.

To determine if you're drinking enough water, a good gauge is the color of your urine. A pale straw color is what you're looking for. Darker urine suggests you should drink more. Another way to tell is the elasticity of your skin: pinch up a fold of skin and release it. If it bounces back fast, you're well hydrated. And if you're checking the pH of your urine daily, acidic urine is a hint that you need to drink more.

Don't drink more than 4 ounces of fluids with any given meal, so that your digestive juices have time to do their work. My typical recommendation is to drink water up to twenty minutes before you eat, then have 4 ounces of fluid with your meal, and wait one to two hours afterward to drink more.

The 16-Day Meal Plan

Feel free to follow this plan exactly as written, or substitute any lunch and dinner with do-it-yourself meals you create based on the food lists. I've also given examples of when you can enjoy leftovers too, so as not to waste food. This meal plan is a guideline only. The recipes begin on page 203.

DAY	MORNING ROUTINE	LUNCH	DINNER
Day 1	Alkalinizing Detox Beverage **or** Mighty Maca Plus drink Coffee or tea with 1 teaspoon to 1 tablespoon MCT oil or coconut oil	*Smoked Salmon and Avocado Salad*	*Garden Harvest Beef Stew* ½ cup cubed mango or papaya, or 1 pineapple ring **or** 1 serving *Mango Coconut Sorbet*
Day 2	Alkalinizing Detox Beverage **or** Mighty Maca Plus drink Coffee or tea with 1 teaspoon to 1 tablespoon MCT oil or coconut oil	Leftover *Smoked Salmon and Avocado Salad* **or** *Spiced Lime Taco Salad*	Leftover *Garden Harvest Beef Stew* **or** *Curry Skillet Chicken with Coconut Cilantro Sauce and Cauli-Rice* ½ cup cubed mango or papaya, or 1 pineapple ring **or** 1 serving *Mango Coconut Sorbet*

(continued)

DAY	MORNING ROUTINE	LUNCH	DINNER
Day 3	Alkalinizing Detox Beverage **or** Mighty Maca Plus drink Coffee or tea with 1 teaspoon to 1 tablespoon MCT oil or coconut oil	Leftover *Spiced Lime Taco Salad* **or** *Farmer's Market Bowl*	Leftover *Curry Skillet Chicken with Coconut Cilantro Sauce and Cauli-Rice* **or** *Fish Tacos with Avocado Salsa and Broccoli Slaw* ½ cup cubed mango or papaya **or** 1 serving *Pineapple Lime Granita*
Day 4	Alkalinizing Detox Beverage **or** Mighty Maca Plus drink Coffee or tea with 1 teaspoon to 1 tablespoon MCT oil or coconut oil	Leftover *Farmer's Market Bowl* **or** *Golden Chicken Thai Salad*	Leftover *Fish Tacos with Avocado Salsa and Broccoli Slaw* **or** *Sheet Pan Herby Chicken with Cruciferous Veggies* ½ cup cubed mango or papaya **or** 1 serving *Pineapple Lime Granita*
Day 5	Alkalinizing Detox Beverage **or** Mighty Maca Plus drink Coffee or tea with 1 teaspoon to 1 tablespoon MCT oil or coconut oil	Leftover *Golden Chicken Thai Salad* **or** *Mediterranean Burger*	Leftover *Sheet Pan Herby Chicken with Cruciferous Veggies* **or** *Spiced Halibut with Crunchy Citrus Salad* ½ cup cubed mango or papaya, or 1 pineapple ring **or** 1 serving *Mango Coconut Sorbet*

DAY	MORNING ROUTINE	LUNCH	DINNER
Day 6	Alkalinizing Detox Beverage **or** Mighty Maca Plus drink Coffee or tea with 1 teaspoon to 1 tablespoon MCT oil or coconut oil	Leftover *Mediterranean Burger* **or** *Zoodle Chicken Pad Thai*	Leftover *Spiced Halibut with Crunchy Citrus Salad* **or** *Lemon Poached Fish with Garlicky Beet Greens* ½ cup cubed mango or papaya, or 1 pineapple ring **or** 1 serving *Mango Coconut Sorbet*
Day 7	Alkalinizing Detox Beverage **or** Mighty Maca Plus drink Coffee or tea with 1 teaspoon to 1 tablespoon MCT oil or coconut oil	Leftover *Zoodle Chicken Pad Thai* **or** *Salmon Salad with Creamy Lemon Dill Dressing*	Leftover *Lemon Poached Fish with Garlicky Beet Greens* **or** *Turmeric Meatballs with Parsley and Sprouts Slaw* ½ cup cubed mango or papaya **or** 1 serving *Pineapple Lime Granita*
Day 8	Alkalinizing Detox Beverage **or** Mighty Maca Plus drink Coffee or tea with 1 teaspoon to 1 tablespoon MCT oil or coconut oil	Leftover *Salmon Salad with Creamy Lemon Dill Dressing* **or** *30-Minute Keto-Green Soup*	Leftover *Turmeric Meatballs with Parsley and Sprouts Slaw* **or** *Chinese Cashew Chicken Lettuce Wraps* ½ cup cubed mango or papaya **or** 1 serving *Pineapple Lime Granita*

(continued)

DAY	MORNING ROUTINE	LUNCH	DINNER
Day 9	Alkalinizing Detox Beverage **or** Mighty Maca Plus drink Coffee or tea with 1 teaspoon to 1 tablespoon MCT oil or coconut oil	Leftover *30-Minute Keto-Green Soup* **or** *Korean Beef and Cabbage*	Leftover *Chinese Cashew Chicken Lettuce Wraps* ½ cup cubed mango or papaya, or 1 pineapple ring **or** 1 serving *Mango Coconut Sorbet*
Day 10	Alkalinizing Detox Beverage **or** Mighty Maca Plus drink Coffee or tea with 1 teaspoon to 1 tablespoon MCT oil or coconut oil	Leftover *Chinese Cashew Chicken Lettuce Wraps* **or** *Skillet Garlic Chicken and Greens*	Leftover *Korean Beef and Cabbage* **or** *Almond-Crusted Chicken Tenders with Cabbage Lime Slaw* ½ cup cubed mango or papaya, or 1 pineapple ring **or** 1 serving *Mango Coconut Sorbet*
Day 11	Alkalinizing Detox Beverage **or** Mighty Maca Plus drink Coffee or tea with 1 teaspoon to 1 tablespoon MCT oil or coconut oil	Leftover *Skillet Garlic Chicken and Greens* **or** *Keto-Green Crudités with Chipotle Cashew Dip*	Leftover *Almond-Crusted Chicken Tenders with Cabbage Lime Slaw* **or** *Ginger Salmon with Crispy Skin and Cruciferous Stir-Fry* ½ cup cubed mango or papaya **or** 1 serving *Pineapple Lime Granita*

DAY	MORNING ROUTINE	LUNCH	DINNER
Day 12	Alkalinizing Detox Beverage **or** Mighty Maca Plus drink Coffee or tea with 1 teaspoon to 1 tablespoon MCT oil or coconut oil	Leftover *Keto-Green Crudités with Chipotle Cashew Dip* **or** *Crunchy Summer Slaw with Halibut*	Leftover *Ginger Salmon with Crispy Skin and Cruciferous Stir-Fry* **or** *One-Pot Roasted Chicken and Veggies with Caramelized Lemons* ½ cup cubed mango or papaya **or** 1 serving *Pineapple Lime Granita*
Day 13	Alkalinizing Detox Beverage **or** Mighty Maca Plus drink Coffee or tea with 1 teaspoon to 1 tablespoon MCT oil or coconut oil	Leftover *Crunchy Summer Slaw with Halibut* **or** *Beef and Cruciferous Tacos with Avocado Lime Crema*	Leftover *One-Pot Roasted Chicken and Veggies with Caramelized Lemons* **or** *Garlic Lime Meatballs with Kimchi Fried Cauli-Rice* ½ cup cubed mango or papaya, or 1 pineapple ring **or** 1 serving *Mango Coconut Sorbet*
Day 14	Alkalinizing Detox Beverage **or** Mighty Maca Plus drink Coffee or tea with 1 teaspoon to 1 tablespoon MCT oil or coconut oil	Leftover *Beef and Cruciferous Tacos with Avocado Lime Crema* **or** *Lemon Pepper Chicken with Brussels Sprouts Slaw*	Leftover *Garlic Lime Meatballs with Kimchi Fried Cauli-Rice* **or** *Not Your Mama's Cabbage Soup* ½ cup cubed mango or papaya **or** 1 serving *Pineapple Lime Granita*

(continued)

DAY	MORNING ROUTINE	LUNCH	DINNER
Day 15	Alkalinizing Detox Beverage **or** Mighty Maca Plus drink Coffee or tea with 1 teaspoon to 1 tablespoon MCT oil or coconut oil	Leftover *Lemon Pepper Chicken with Brussels Sprouts Slaw* **or** *Roasted Cabbage with Chicken and Shallots*	Leftover *Not Your Mama's Cabbage Soup* **or** *Garlic Roasted Cabbage and Chicken* ½ cup cubed mango or papaya **or** 1 serving *Pineapple Lime Granita*
Day 16	Alkalinizing Detox Beverage **or** Mighty Maca Plus drink Coffee or tea with 1 teaspoon to 1 tablespoon MCT oil or coconut oil	Leftover *Roasted Cabbage with Chicken and Shallots* **or** *Egg Hand Salad*	*Coconut Ginger Chicken with Cilantro Cauli-Rice* **or** *Cabbage Roll Stew* ½ cup cubed mango or papaya, or 1 pineapple ring **or** 1 serving *Mango Coconut Sorbet*

Get ready to love what you'll see in the mirror as pounds and inches come off in all the right places. You'll start to feel so much better in no time at all after following this safe, simple, scientific approach to weight loss and hormone balance. It's just sixteen days, but it will be among the most rewarding sixteen days you've ever spent losing weight.

Chapter 6

The Vegan Keto-Green 16 Diet Plan

. . . .

Many people are opting to eat less meat these days—whether to improve their health, the environment, animal welfare, or the economy. If you're among them, I've got a plant-based version of my fat-burning and hormone-fixing Keto-Green 16 plan just for you. It's designed so that vegans and all plant-based eaters can join the Keto-Green movement.

If you're already following a plant-based diet, this plan will upgrade your nutrition to include higher amounts of fat, along with plenty of alkalinizing foods to balance blood sugar, improve metabolism, and drop weight. Vegetarians of all types can join in too. So can omnivores who'd like to fast from animal products—a strategy that I support and feel is very beneficial. I recommend taking a break from animal foods at least twice a year, in two different sixteen-day cycles.

You might be asking yourself how it's possible to combine a ketogenic diet with a vegan one. Wouldn't that be really hard or overly restrictive? Well, I'm here to show you exactly how to do this, using whole, alkalinizing plant-based foods. Not only can it be done, but it can be delicious and help you to move the needle on your health in a dramatic way!

As a plant-based eater, in some ways you'll have an easier time getting alkaline, because whole plant foods, especially greens, are really supportive of this. However, sometimes it takes a little more care to get into ketosis because plant foods are also naturally higher in carbohydrates. For example, when you swap out grass-fed beef in a keto recipe for tofu, that soy-based food will provide some carbs, whereas the beef does not. Just be patient, though, and you'll get there.

The Macros on the Vegan Keto-Green 16 Diet

At its core, this plan is a 100-percent plant-based diet, designed to help you achieve the right daily balance of protein, carbohydrates, and fat. Like the Keto-Green 16 plan, this version focuses on reducing carbs that put you on a roller coaster of insulin spikes and restrict your body's ability to burn fat. This allows you to regulate your insulin levels and get your body to use its fat stores for energy, and so it results in weight loss. It also supports ketosis, alkalinity, and hormone balancing. Plus it alleviates cravings.

For protein at meals, you'll substitute black soybeans, white beans, or chickpeas for beef, fish, and chicken. Beans are one of nature's superfoods. They are full of protein, fiber, and various vitamins and minerals. What's more, they have many health benefits, including a reduction in cancer risk.

Yes, beans are higher in carbs than animal protein, so you have to be careful in terms of the quantity of beans you eat. The beans I've included are among the lower-carb types. Black soybeans, for example, contain only 8 grams of carbs per cup. Chickpeas are slightly higher in carbs, at 34 carbs per cup. Finally, white beans hold 45 grams of carbs per cup, so you have to be a little stingy on how much of these you eat. The guidelines that follow will help you.

For fat-burning, you can reach and maintain ketosis by relying on high-fat, plant-based fats such as coconut oil, olive oil, avocados, avocado oil, seeds, and nuts.

I've included several vegan recipes in the recipe section.

The Vegan Keto-Green 16 Food List

Your food list is similar to the regular plan, with the exception of animal foods. Choose from these sixteen foods and food groups:

1. Black soybeans (protein)*

2. White beans (protein)*

3. Chickpeas (protein)*

4. Dark leafy greens, raw or cooked (alkalinizing vegetables such as spinach, kale, beet greens, bok choy, Swiss chard, mustard greens, collard greens, arugula, and lettuces of all varieties)

5. Sprouts, raw (alkalinizing vegetable)

6. Cabbage, cooked or raw (alkalinizing vegetable)

7. Cruciferous vegetables such as broccoli and cauliflower, cooked or raw (alkalinizing vegetables)

8. Onion/garlic (alkalinizing vegetables)

9. Lemons or limes, freshly juiced to add to the morning Alkalinizing Detox Beverage or to season vegetables (alkalinizing fruits)

10. MCT oil or coconut oil (fats)

11. Olive oil, avocado oil, or coconut ghee

12. Nuts and seeds—Brazil nuts, almonds, hazelnuts, pili nuts, sunflower seeds, and hemp seeds (fats)

13. Avocado (fat)

14. Sauerkraut, kimchi, and pickled ginger (digestive support vegetables)

---

* You may replace beans with non-GMO tofu or tempeh (protein)

15. Pineapple, mango, or papaya (digestive support fruits)

16. *Keto Alkaline Broth,* page 221 (alkalinizing support food)

When Keto-Green Meets Vegan: The Upside

Both the Keto-Green 16 diet and its vegan counterpart can benefit your health in similar ways. For example, we know from research that vegans tend to weigh less than non-vegans. We also know that ketogenic diets produce significant and sustainable weight loss. Combine the two into a vegan keto-alkalinizing plan, and you're in super fat-burning territory. Both the keto diet and a vegan diet are well known for their effectiveness not only in weight loss but also in blood sugar and insulin control and reduction of heart disease and diabetes risk factors.

As for hormone-balancing, the Vegan Keto-Green 16 approach pulls out the stops here too. You'll be eating lots of cruciferous vegetables such as broccoli, cabbage, cauliflower, bok choy, and Brussels sprouts—all of which contain high amounts of glucosinolates. These are natural detoxifying substances that help usher harmful estrogens from the body.

Chewing, chopping, or even blending these vegetables activates an enzyme that converts them into indole-3-carbinol, which enhances the liver's detoxification powers. It can then efficiently eliminate toxins and unhealthy hormones from the body for a balancing effect.

This plan is also rich in fiber, especially compared to a more standard ketogenic diet. The fiber helps balance blood sugar and produce satiety after meals. Fiber is helpful for regularity and preventing the constipation that sometimes occurs as dietary fat increases. Fiber creates a healthy microbiome well populated with friendly gut bacteria, which in turn supports weight control, immunity, and hormone balance.

The Vegan Keto-Green 16 approach is also extremely high in phytonutrients (plant compounds) that offer a host of protective benefits to the body. Phytonutrients such as carotenoids, flavonoids, and others can play diverse and healing roles in the body. Most notably, they act as antioxidants protecting cells from free-radical damage and decreasing inflammation and chronic disease. Phytonutrients are associated with all of the colors that you find in whole produce, so eat a rainbow to take full advantage of this plan.

You'll be enjoying avocados on this version too. They are packed with beta-sitosterol, a natural substance that helps regulate and balance cortisol and restore low DHEA.

Foods that are fermented, such as sauerkraut and kimchi, deliver beneficial probiotics to your digestive system, helping to boost its population of friendly bacteria. Foods rich in "prebiotics," such as onions and garlic, are important too, because these are foods that friendly bacteria feed on. All of these actions create a healthy gut and a healthy body.

So if you're a dedicated plant-based eater who wants to lose weight and inches and to get your hormones back in balance, the Vegan Keto-Green 16 diet is the right course of action.

BENEFITS OF GOING VEGAN KETO-GREEN

- Improved bone health

- Improved cardiovascular health

- Improved fat-burning

- Maintenance of lean muscle

- Youthfulness

- Prevents magnesium deficiency

- Reduced pain

- Reduced inflammation

- Improved detoxification

- Hormonal balance

- Weight loss

- Enhanced sex drive

- Increased energy

- Improved sleep quality

Building Your Meals

You can create your meals, follow the menu plan exactly, or do a little of both. Here's a simple template for creating vegan lunches and dinners. Also, look for the recipes labeled "Vegan Friendly" in the recipe section.

Upon Awakening

Prepare and drink my Alkalinizing Detox Beverage or Dr. Anna Cabeca Mighty Maca Plus drink, followed by coffee or tea with 1 teaspoon to 1 tablespoon MCT oil or coconut oil, and optional 1 teaspoon coconut ghee.

Lunch (11 A.M.)

Lunch = 1 vegan protein serving + 1 to 2 servings alkalinizing vegetables + 1 to 2 fat servings

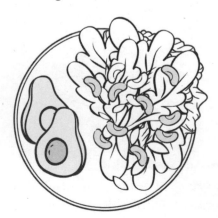

Examples:

- ½ to 1 cup black soybeans + 1 to 2 cups spinach, kale, or beet greens sautéed in 1 tablespoon olive oil or coconut oil or avocado oil + ½ avocado, sliced

- ½ cup chickpeas atop a bed of fresh greens, chopped raw cauliflower, and chopped onions. Sprinkle with 1 tablespoon chopped almonds and toss with 1 tablespoon olive oil and juice from ½ to 1 lemon.

- Any of the vegan lunch recipes provided

- Any of the regular lunch recipes provided, but without fish, chicken, or beef (use beans, tofu, or tempeh instead)

Dinner (finishing by 6 to 7 P.M.)

Dinner = 1 vegan protein serving + 2 servings alkalinizing vegetables + 1 to 2 fat servings + digestive support food

After dinner, take 2 digestive enzyme supplements.

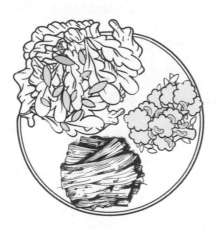

Examples:

- ½ to 1 cup black soybeans + cauliflower rice + side salad with fresh greens and 1 tablespoon chopped nuts tossed with

1 tablespoon olive oil and juice from ½ to 1 lemon + 1 serving of sauerkraut or kimchi

- ¼ to ½ cup white beans atop 1 to 2 cups spinach, kale, or beet greens sautéed in 1 tablespoon olive oil, coconut oil, or avocado oil, followed by ½ cup cubed mango or papaya

- Any of the vegan dinner recipes provided

- Any of the regular dinner recipes provided, but without fish, chicken, or beef (use beans, tofu, or tempeh instead)

Snacking Options

Although I do not recommend snacking, some people need Keto-Green snacks to curb hunger and cravings. If this describes you, feel free to include these snacks from the list of sixteen foods during your eight-hour feeding period:

- ¼ cup nuts

- ½ avocado drizzled with olive oil and sea salt

- A Keto-Green shake or smoothie (pages 204–218)

- 1 cup *Keto Alkaline Broth* (page 221)

- 1 cup raw cruciferous veggies such as broccoli or cauliflower

The Vegan Keto-Green Meal Replacement Option

As with the Keto-Green 16 plan, you may replace any lunch or dinner with a Keto-Green shake or smoothie (pages 204–218), made with the Keto-Green Meal Replacement powder—which is perfect for vegans and vegetarians. If it's hard to meet your protein needs or get enough protein diversity as you progress through this program, this powdered supplement can be your best ally.

You may also have one of these smoothies whenever you feel

you need a little extra fuel. If you are someone who deals with late-night food cravings, drink my Willpower Mama smoothie at 5 P.M. The fat and fiber it contains will fill you up.

Reminders and Guidelines

- Test your urinary pH first thing in the morning (and periodically throughout the day), with the goal of keeping at or above 7.0. The greener the strip, the more alkaline your body. As for ketones, the pinker the strip, the higher your level of ketosis. Record everything.

- Practice intermittent fasting. Remember, you'll finish your dinner by 6 or 7 P.M. each evening, with no food or fluids overnight, with the exception of herbal tea, water, or *Keto Alkaline Broth* (page 221).

  You'll eat your first meal of the day sixteen hours after you finished dinner the previous night—usually at 10 or 11 A.M. If you're a beginner or intermediate, you'll have a shorter fasting window—twelve to thirteen hours for beginners and fourteen to fifteen hours for intermediates—and you can break your fast with a Keto-Green smoothie (pages 204–218).

- Design your Keto-Green vegan plate. On a plate, this means greens and alkalinizing vegetables account for 75 percent of the surface area. Plant proteins make up a palm-size amount, approximately ½ to 1 cup. Then imagine a circle in the center of the plate, which equals approximately ¼ cup healthy fats, such as avocados, nuts, or olive oil. Lunch can also be one of my Keto-Green smoothies.

- Hydrate! With all of this plant fiber and high-fat, low-carb vegan options, it is extremely important to drink enough water each day. My rule of thumb is to drink 60 to 70 ounces of pure water daily (not with meals, to avoid diluting important digestive enzymes).

- Boost your mineral intake. You naturally get a lot of electrolyte minerals from your alkalinizing veggies, but you may benefit from added sea salt and perhaps a magnesium supplement. Another great strategy is to enjoy *Keto Alkaline Broth* (page 221). I suggest several mugs each day, or when you feel hungry.

- Don't forget herbs and spices. Even though they don't contribute many calories or carbs, they do deliver on micronutrients, phytonutrients, and flavor. Plus they can keep daily food choices interesting and diverse.

- Stay in ketosis by restricting your carbohydrate intake to 40 grams per day or less and making sure to eat your allotment of fats.

- Do not eat between meals and do not snack. If you're over forty, snacking can be destructive to your goals. It can cause insulin resistance, weight gain, hot flashes, and inflammation. If you feel hunger pangs during the day, see the snacking options discussed earlier. You can add more healthy fats, oils, and nuts to a green leafy salad as a snack, or enjoy a large cup of *Keto Alkaline Broth* (page 221).

- Be sure to rest when your body is asking you to. Instead of pushing yourself, give yourself time and space to relax into these changes in your body. These actions, along with getting quality sleep, will help you stay alkaline. Epsom salt baths, massage, naps, and gentle walking are all great tools to use as well.

JUMP-START KETOSIS

Sometimes it is a little more challenging for plant-based eaters to get into ketosis. But I have some solutions. If at any time, especially in the beginning, you find it hard to achieve ketosis, try the following:

- Stay with the intermittent fasting protocol.

- Always begin your day with the morning routine of the Alkalinizing Detox Beverage or Mighty Maca Plus drink, followed by coffee or tea with 1 teaspoon to 1 tablespoon MCT oil or coconut oil.

- At lunch, enjoy a Keto-Green shake or smoothie (pages 204–218).

- For dinner, have a large bowl of *Keto Alkaline Broth* (page 221), *Curried Cabbage Keto-Green Soup* (page 239), or *Keto-Green Gazpacho* (page 240).

- Use some additional MCT oil or coconut oil in your coffee, tea, smoothies, or soups.

Implement this strategy for three days in a row. You may use it at any juncture during the sixteen days of the diet.

The 16-Day Meal Plan

Feel free to follow this plan exactly as written, or substitute any lunch or dinner with meals you create based on the food lists. This meal plan is a guideline only.

DAY	MORNING ROUTINE	LUNCH	DINNER
Day 1	Alkalinizing Detox Beverage **or** Mighty Maca Plus drink	*Pineapple Keto-Green Smoothie*	*Curried Cabbage Keto-Green Soup* **or** *Garden Harvest Beef Stew* (replace beef with 1 cup cooked white beans)
		¼ cup macadamia nuts	
	Coffee or tea with 1 teaspoon to 1 tablespoon MCT oil or coconut oil		½ cup cubed mango or papaya **or** 1 serving *Pineapple Lime Granita*
Day 2	Alkalinizing Detox Beverage **or** Mighty Maca Plus drink	Leftover *Curried Cabbage Keto-Green Soup* **or** *Toasted Tempeh Noodle Bowl with Cilantro Lime Greens*	Leftover *Garden Harvest Beef Stew* (replace beef with 1 cup cooked white beans) **or** *Cruciferous Stir-Fry* (replace salmon with 4 ounces tofu or tempeh)
	Coffee or tea with 1 teaspoon to 1 tablespoon MCT oil or coconut oil		½ cup cubed mango or papaya **or** 1 serving *Pineapple Lime Granita*

DAY	MORNING ROUTINE	LUNCH	DINNER
Day 3	Alkalinizing Detox Beverage **or** Mighty Maca Plus drink Coffee or tea with 1 teaspoon to 1 tablespoon MCT oil or coconut oil	*Yogurt Bowl with Keto-Green-ola*	*White "Keto-ney Bean" Stir-Fry* **or** Leftover *Cruciferous Stir-Fry* (replace salmon with 4 ounces tofu or tempeh) ½ cup cubed mango or papaya, or 1 ring pineapple **or** 1 serving *Mango Coconut Sorbet*
Day 4	Alkalinizing Detox Beverage **or** Mighty Maca Plus drink Coffee or tea with 1 teaspoon to 1 tablespoon MCT oil or coconut oil	*Keto-Green Raw Wraps with Zucchini–White Bean Hummus*	Cauliflower crust pizza topped with non-starchy veggies **or** *Fish Tacos with Avocado Salsa and Broccoli Slaw* (replace fish with ½ cup black soybeans) ½ cup cubed mango or papaya, or 1 ring pineapple **or** 1 serving *Mango Coconut Sorbet*

(continued)

DAY	MORNING ROUTINE	LUNCH	DINNER
Day 5	Alkalinizing Detox Beverage **or** Mighty Maca Plus drink Coffee or tea with 1 teaspoon to 1 tablespoon MCT oil or coconut oil	*Farmer's Market Bowl* (replace chicken with black soybeans or chickpeas)	*Leftover Fish Tacos with Avocado Salsa and Broccoli Slaw* (replace fish with ½ cup black soybeans) **or** *Cauliflower "Gnocchi" with Pesto and White Beans* ½ cup cubed mango or papaya **or** 1 serving *Pineapple Lime Granita*
Day 6	Alkalinizing Detox Beverage **or** Mighty Maca Plus drink Coffee or tea with 1 teaspoon to 1 tablespoon MCT oil or coconut oil	*Keto-Green Pâté Endive Boats*	Cauliflower crust pizza topped with non-starchy veggies **or** Leftover *Fish Tacos with Avocado Salsa and Broccoli Slaw* (replace fish with ½ cup black soybeans) ½ cup cubed mango or papaya **or** 1 serving *Pineapple Lime Granita*
Day 7	Alkalinizing Detox Beverage **or** Mighty Maca Plus drink Coffee or tea with 1 teaspoon to 1 tablespoon MCT oil or coconut oil	*Buddha Bowl*	*Cashew Curry with Vegetables over Keto "Rice"* ½ cup cubed mango or papaya, or 1 ring pineapple **or** 1 serving of *Mango Coconut Sorbet*

DAY	MORNING ROUTINE	LUNCH	DINNER
Day 8	Alkalinizing Detox Beverage **or** Mighty Maca Plus drink Coffee or tea with 1 teaspoon to 1 tablespoon MCT oil or coconut oil	Leftover *Cashew Curry with Vegetables over Keto "Rice"*	*Zucchini Noodles with Walnut Romesco Sauce* ½ cup cubed mango or papaya, or 1 ring pineapple **or** 1 serving *Mango Coconut Sorbet*
Day 9	Alkalinizing Detox Beverage **or** Mighty Maca Plus drink Coffee or tea with 1 teaspoon to 1 tablespoon MCT oil or coconut oil	Leftover *Zucchini Noodles with Walnut Romesco Sauce*	*Massaged Kale Salad with Almond Miso Dressing* ½ cup cubed mango or papaya **or** 1 serving *Pineapple Lime Granita*
Day 10	Alkalinizing Detox Beverage **or** Mighty Maca Plus drink Coffee or tea with 1 teaspoon to 1 tablespoon MCT oil or coconut oil	*Buddha Bowl*	*White "Keto-ney Bean" Stir-Fry* ½ cup cubed mango or papaya **or** 1 serving *Pineapple Lime Granita*
Day 11	Alkalinizing Detox Beverage **or** Mighty Maca Plus drink Coffee or tea with 1 teaspoon to 1 tablespoon MCT oil or coconut oil	Leftover *White "Keto-ney Bean" Stir-Fry*	*Zoodle Chicken Pad Thai* (replace chicken with 4 ounces tofu or tempeh) ½ cup cubed mango or papaya, or 1 ring pineapple **or** 1 serving *Mango Coconut Sorbet*

(continued)

DAY	MORNING ROUTINE	LUNCH	DINNER
Day 12	Alkalinizing Detox Beverage **or** Mighty Maca Plus drink Coffee or tea with 1 teaspoon to 1 tablespoon MCT oil or coconut oil	Leftover *Zoodle Chicken Pad Thai* (replace chicken with 4 ounces tofu or tempeh)	*Spiced Halibut with Crunchy Citrus Salad* (replace halibut with ½ cup chickpeas) ½ cup cubed mango or papaya **or** 1 serving *Mango Coconut Sorbet*
Day 13	Alkalinizing Detox Beverage **or** Mighty Maca Plus drink Coffee or tea with 1 teaspoon to 1 tablespoon MCT oil or coconut oil	*Pineapple Keto-Green Smoothie* ¼ cup macadamia nuts **or** Leftover *Spiced Halibut with Crunchy Citrus Salad* (replace halibut with ½ cup chickpeas)	*Curried Cabbage Keto-Green Soup* ½ cup cubed mango or papaya
Day 14	Alkalinizing Detox Beverage **or** Mighty Maca Plus drink Coffee or tea with 1 teaspoon to 1 tablespoon MCT oil or coconut oil	Leftover *Curried Cabbage Keto-Green Soup*	*Chinese Cashew Chicken Lettuce Wraps* (replace chicken with ½ cup chickpeas) ½ cup cubed mango or papaya **or** 1 serving *Pineapple Lime Granita*

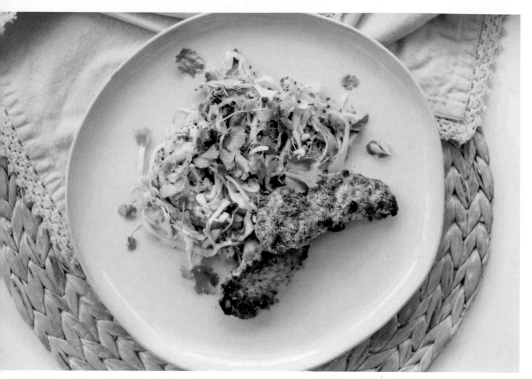

Almond-Crusted Chicken Tenders with Cabbage Lime Slaw (page 249)

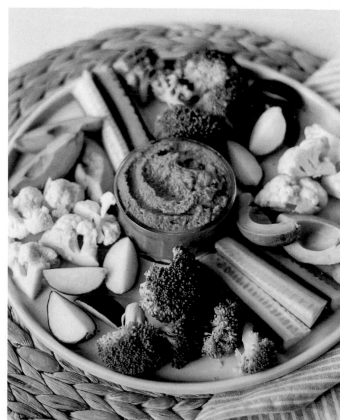

*Keto-Green Crudités
with Chipotle Cashew Dip
(page 227)*

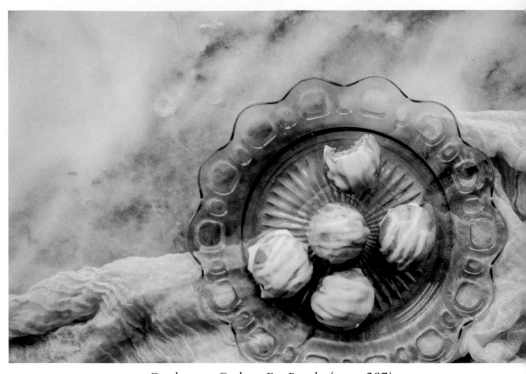

Cardamom Cashew Fat Bombs (page 287)

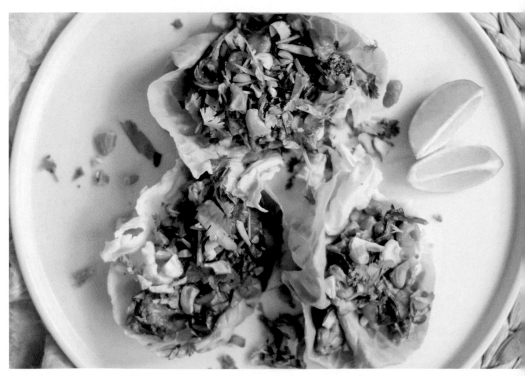

Chinese Cashew Chicken Lettuce Wraps (page 262)

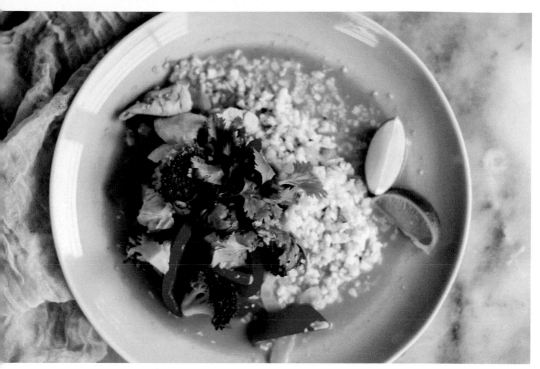

Coconut Ginger Chicken with Cilantro Cauli-Rice (page 268)

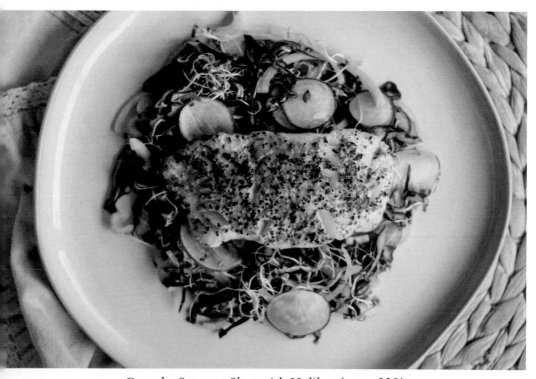

Crunchy Summer Slaw with Halibut (page 229)

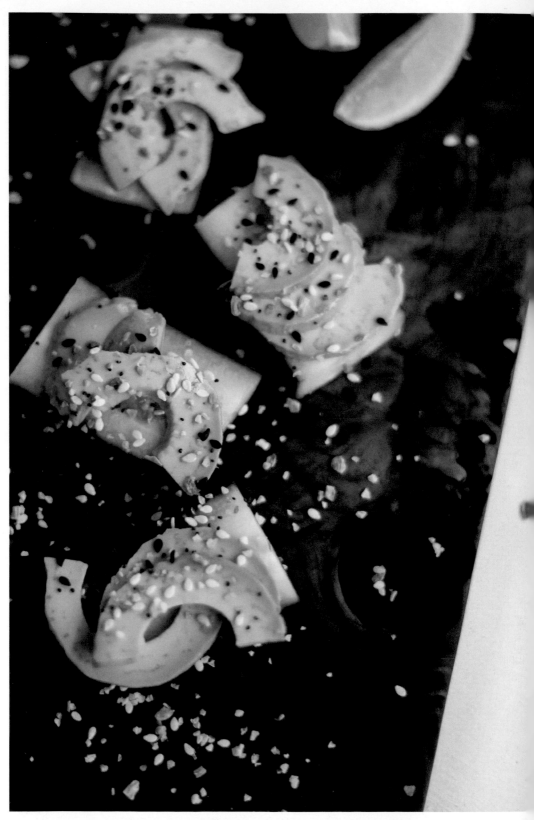

Cucumber Avocado Open-Faced "Sandwiches" (page 282)

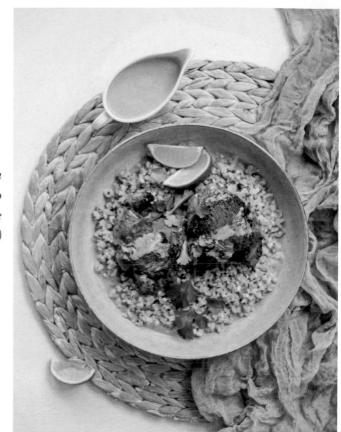

Curry Skillet Chicken with Coconut Cilantro Sauce and Cauli-Rice (page 252)

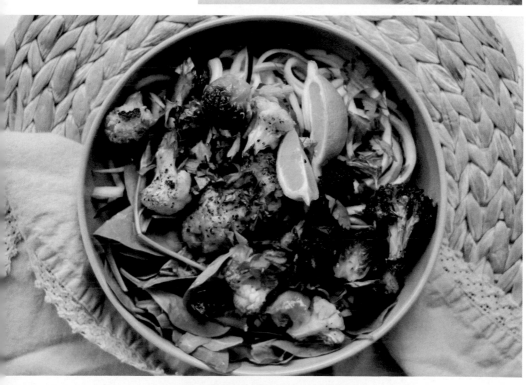

Farmer's Market Bowl (page 225)

Garden Harvest
Beef Stew (page 251)

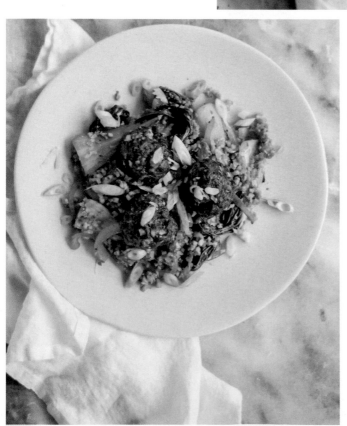

Garlic Lime Meatballs with
Kimchi Fried Cauli-Rice
(page 259)

Garlic Roasted Cabbage and Chicken (page 265)

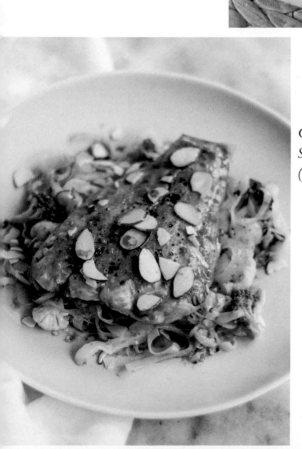

Ginger Salmon with Crispy Skin and Cruciferous Stir-Fry (page 254)

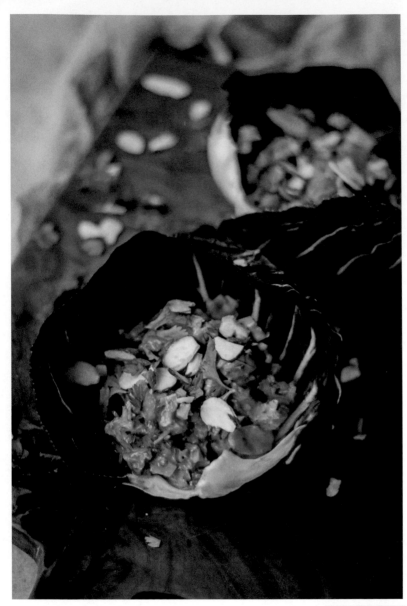

Golden Chicken Thai Salad (page 230)

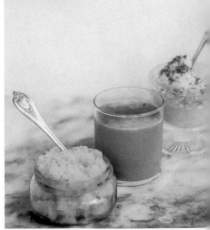

*Pineapple Lime Granita (page 288),
Tropical Turmeric Milkshake (page 218),
and Mango Coconut Sorbet (page 286)*

DAY	MORNING ROUTINE	LUNCH	DINNER
Day 15	Alkalinizing Detox Beverage **or** Mighty Maca Plus drink Coffee or tea with 1 teaspoon to 1 tablespoon MCT oil or coconut oil	*Chocolate Keto-Green Smoothie*	Leftover *Chinese Cashew Chicken Lettuce Wraps* (replace chicken with ½ cup chickpeas) ½ cup cubed mango or papaya, or 1 ring pineapple **or** 1 serving *Mango Coconut Sorbet*
Day 16	Alkalinizing Detox Beverage **or** Mighty Maca Plus drink Coffee or tea with 1 teaspoon to 1 tablespoon MCT oil or coconut oil	*Keto Alkaline Broth* **or** *Keto-Green smoothie*	*Keto-Green Gazpacho* ½ cup cubed mango or papaya, or 1 ring pineapple **or** 1 serving *Mango Coconut Sorbet*

Fill in Nutritional Gaps

One possible obstacle to overcome with Vegan Keto-Green 16 is that you may need to fill in some nutritional gaps for key nutrients if you're not getting enough (or absorbing enough) from your diet. Here are some strategies to consider.

Vitamin A

Vitamin A is important for immunity, cell growth, and vision. It generally comes in the preformed (active form) from animal foods, and as carotenoids, such as beta-carotene, from plants.

Your body can convert beta-carotene from Keto-Green foods like kale into vitamin A, but the process isn't that efficient, and some people may have genetic variations that make it even less so.

Ways to increase vitamin A:

- Supplement beta-carotene and/or preformed vitamin A.

- Consider taking a tablespoon of cod liver oil if you can (although cod liver oil is not vegan).

Vitamin D

Vitamin D is important for bone health and immunity, and acts more like a hormone in the body affecting every cell. In my practice, I saw vitamin D deficiencies all the time, in vegetarians and omnivores alike.

We get vitamin D from exposing ourselves to sunlight (without sunscreen) as long as we are at the right latitude and the right time of year. Vitamin D2, the plant version, is found in mushrooms.

Ways to increase vitamin D:

- Increase sunlight exposure as appropriate for your body.

- Supplement with vitamin D. Have your doctor check your vitamin D levels and then dose accordingly.

Iron

Iron is the mineral in your red blood cells that carries oxygen to every part of the body. Without enough iron, anemia can occur, leaving you feeling tired and with a sluggish metabolism. There are two types of iron in food. Heme iron is better absorbed and is found in animal foods, mainly muscle meats and organ meats. Non-heme iron is found in plant foods such as leafy greens and sunflower seeds.

Ways to increase your iron:

- Pair your Vegan Keto-Green iron sources along with vitamin C to help increase iron absorption. Add lemon juice to sautéed greens or over salads, for example.

- Increase herbal teas, such as nettles, that provide iron and other minerals.

Zinc

This mineral is vital for the immune system, building hormones (especially testosterone), and protecting the gut. It is found mostly in animal foods, so vegans are often deficient.

To increase your intake of this mineral, I recommend supplementation of 30–60 mg zinc daily.

Omega-3 Fats

Omega-3 fats are important for cellular structure, cellular communication, brain health, and reducing inflammation. The body has the ability to turn some of the alpha-linolenic acid we get from plant foods like flax, hemp seeds, and walnuts into the bigger molecules of EPA and DHA that are incredibly important for health. However, like we discussed with vitamin A, this conversion process isn't great, and some of us are worse at it than others.

Ways to increase EPA and DHA:

- Increase flaxseeds, walnuts, hemp seeds, and chia seeds. Use flaxseed oil or walnut oil, but don't heat it, and store in the fridge to protect the fragile fats. (Avoid seeds, however, if you have digestive problems; they can lodge in your large intestine.)

- Supplement with an algae-based omega-3 supplement or cod liver oil (which is not vegan).

Vitamin B12

Vitamin B12 is important for cell formation (including blood cells) and gene expression (the overall process of making proteins with the information coded in DNA). When vitamin B12 is in short supply, you might feel pretty fatigued. B12 is found primarily in animal foods, making it important for vegetarians and vegans to pay attention to.

Ways to increase vitamin B12:

- Add nutritional yeast to daily meals as a source of B12 and other B vitamins.

- Consider a multivitamin or B complex for supplemental support.

I've got more information for you on supplementation in Chapter 7. Don't miss it!

Lots of Variety for Lots of Success

There are so many delicious plant foods and recipes that are low in carbs and high in fat and protein that you should have no problem losing pounds and inches and feeling great on this plan. It's a myth that vegans and other plant-based eaters can't go keto or low-carb. They most certainly can!

Chapter 7

Weight-Control Supplements That Really Work

As I've shared, I struggled with my weight for a long time, eventually weighing more than 240 pounds. Way before then, however, I was a chubby child. In my teens, I started dieting—the beginning of years and years as a yo-yo dieter, with my weight swinging dramatically from highs to lows and back again.

My career as a solo OB/GYN meant long hours, no time for myself, and a nutrient-poor diet of too much caffeine and one or two grab-and-go meals a day (that's *not* the way to fast!). All of this, plus my chaotic schedule, was self-defeating and did nothing positive for my body. Mine was a textbook case of hormone imbalance, with unhealthy doses of stress, hidden food sensitivities, too many carbs, and not enough self-care.

Determined to lead a healthier life, I changed my diet to an earlier version of my Keto-Green plan; since perfecting it for patients and clients, I now follow what I've given you in this book. My goal was to restore and rebalance my hormones so that I could reach the healthiest possible weight. I was successful, and afterward I decided that hormone chaos would never again rule my weight and waistline. I know you want the same results.

Part of the strategy I devised to achieve a sexy, happy, and healthy state involved nutritional supplementation, with the emphasis on those supplements that address weight and our weight-control hormones. The supplements I recommend will help restore your hormones and give you the physical, mental, and emotional energy to move forward positively toward your happy weight.

If you really want to lose weight and feel better for the long term—and stay there—you've got to go a little deeper with your nutrition. To accomplish this, I suggest adding herbal, hormonal, and nutritional supplements to the Keto-Green 16 diet.

A common but important question that I get asked all the time is why we need to supplement if we eat a nutrient-rich diet. Fast disappearing from nutritional dogma is the notion that food can give us everything we need. Unlike the native cultures I observed while traveling around the world, we're living in times of more stress and tension; we're indoors more often than not and so we don't get vitamin D and energy from the sun; we're more sedentary than ever, and our foods are not as fresh as they used to be. We live in a hazardous, hormone-depleting environment and an unnatural landscape. Therefore, the answer is yes—I do think we require heroic countermeasures in the form of supplements to balance our hormones, help control our weight, and enhance our health and longevity.

Because of these realities and what I learned from healers all over the world, I've spent a lot of time studying and researching the quality, bioavailability, sustainability, and efficacy of various supplements and am therefore very particular about what I recommend. And so I've identified a number of supplements that strike at the very core of hormone imbalance and the weight it produces. They are remarkably safe and easily obtainable from your health food store, pharmacy, or online.

I'm not saying, however, that if you pop some of these, you'll magically become thin and fit. Not at all. You have to use them in conjunction with Keto-Green eating, its lifestyle, and exercise for the very best results. Nor do you have to take supplements to be successful. However, I know from working with thousands of men and women that you will feel better if you choose to supplement.

The irreversible reality is that most of our hor away, and supplementing, along with this diet, c mental difference in your life, especially for those fifty.

So why not take action now, replenish your vitality, your youthful figure? Here are my recommendations you started.

Vitamin Supplements

A Multivitamin/mineral

Vitamins and minerals are required for nearly all metabolic and developmental bodily processes, and they are instrumental as nutritional insurance. Although someone's diet might be well planned, it's not always possible for most people to select foods that have the recommended amounts of all essential nutrients. Even relatively minor shortfalls of a nutrient can cause health problems. That's why it's so important to bridge nutrient gaps with vitamins and minerals.

In 2014, the *Nutrition Journal* published an extensive review, pointing out that people who take vitamins and minerals delay the onset and severity of serious diseases—and in some cases slash the odds of getting them. These include cancer, heart disease, and brain and cognitive problems, among others. The article further pointed out that death rates are lower among regular vitamin takers (both men and women), especially if they supplement with vitamins A, C, or E in addition to their multiple.

Without supplementation, many people will suffer nutrient deficiencies that put them at a hormonal disadvantage. If your body is lacking in zinc, iron, and B vitamins, for example, you may have signs of a hormonal imbalance such as polycystic ovary syndrome or infertility, or you could miscarry. The body depends on an intricate balance of nutrients in order to get the reproductive processes working well.

One reason many people still hold out on taking a multivitamin is that there are many types on the market, and they are not all the same; it's confusing! The ones I recommend have a multivitamin/mineral blend featuring activated vitamins, including folate as 5-MTHF (5-methyltetrahydrofolate), and Albion chelated mineral complexes, because these are well absorbed.

I also suggest that you choose a multivitamin/mineral supplement that includes bioavailable B vitamins. Recent evidence suggests that dietary intake of the B vitamins, including B6, B9, and B12, helps regulate the stress hormone cortisol, which in excess drives the body to store fat, as well as creating other metabolic havoc. The B vitamins do their job by supporting the function of your adrenal glands, which secrete cortisol and other stress hormones. B vitamins can be stolen away by adrenal stress and high cortisol levels.

Found in animal foods, vitamin B12 is particularly vulnerable. A deficiency can lead to decreased estrogen and progesterone, along with increased cortisol levels. It is the single most important nutrient affected by aging and starts its downhill descent by midlife — which is why supplementation is essential.

When your adrenals are balanced — thanks to the B vitamins and other nutrients — your weight can return to a healthy level.

Recommended dosage: I prefer multivitamin/minerals that you take in divided doses — 2 tablets daily, 1 in the morning and 1 in the evening (preferably with food). This infuses your body with nutrients throughout the day. If you prefer to take a once-a-day formula, that is fine too.

Extra Vitamin C

Most multivitamins contain vitamin C; however, the amount is not enough to obtain the therapeutic amounts of the vitamin shown in research to help prevent heart disease and boost immune function.

Vitamin C is an antioxidant and is everyone's favorite supplement, most linked to fighting the common cold, combating cancer, and supporting the formation of skin-tightening collagen. There is even solid proof that vitamin C can add years to your life.

Hormonally, vitamin C offers wholesale protection against excess levels of cortisol. In one quite remarkable study, German researchers put 120 people in a surefire stressful situation: public speaking combined with solving a math problem. Half of the participants supplemented with 1,000 mg of vitamin C; the other half did not. Signs of stress—elevated cortisol and blood pressure—soared in the non-supplementers, while those who took the vitamin did not have such an acute response and felt less stressed while going through the tasks.

Vitamin C's ability to rein in cortisol, support the adrenal glands, and enhance liver detoxification are some of the chief reasons I recommend it as a supplement for the Keto-Green 16 plan. This nutrient is also important for boosting immunity and protecting cells from disease.

Recommended dosage: Start with a daily dose of 500 to 2,000 mg, taken any time of the day. As a gynecologist, let me add that taking 2,000 to 4,000 mg daily helps prevent urinary tract infections.

Vitamin D

We need more vitamin D; unfortunately, multivitamins quite often do not contain enough of this vitamin to meet our needs, nor to optimize our vitamin D blood levels. Technically a pro-hormone, not a vitamin, vitamin D gets a lot of attention for its effect on health. It also turns out that it is a special-forces agent in the war against obesity. As a fat burner, it appears to work in four important ways. First, when you have optimal levels of vitamin D, your body produces more leptin, the hormone that sends a message to your brain that you're full and don't need to eat anymore. Second, with an ample supply of vitamin D, your fat cells resist making and storing fat. Third, vitamin D may work with calcium to reduce the overproduction of cortisol, that pesky stress hormone which triggers the storage of belly fat. Finally, vitamin D is essential for hormones to work together properly, especially progesterone and oxytocin.

Vitamin D is naturally found in some foods, such as fatty fish, and is synthesized in the body when your skin is exposed to sunlight for even just ten minutes a day.

Even so, most people don't get enough vitamin D due to living in more northerly climates or not eating enough vitamin-D-rich foods — which is why supplementation is important.

There are two types of vitamin D: vitamin D2 and vitamin D3. Both can be taken in supplement form. Vitamin D3 is produced in response to sun exposure and is found in animal products, whereas vitamin D2 occurs in plants. Vitamin D3 has been found to increase blood levels significantly more than D2.

However, it's also possible — although rare — for this vitamin to build up and reach toxic levels in your body. It is recommended that you do not exceed an upper limit of 10,000 international units (IU) per day of any type of vitamin D.

Recommended dosage: It's important that you get some sun daily, especially in the morning and early evening (when the rays aren't as damaging) so that your skin and eyes are exposed to sunlight.

I recommend that you have your vitamin D levels checked via a blood test, then supplement or get sun as needed. (A normal reading is between 50 and 80 ng/mL.)

The Institute of Medicine advises 600 IU of vitamin D a day. You may need more, so discuss dosage with your physician. Look for a supplement that also contains vitamin K2, which helps the body better absorb vitamin D. I typically recommend 2,000 to 5,000 IU of vitamin D3 daily, with up to 45 mcg of vitamin K2.

Herbal Supplements

Black Cohosh

Discovered by Native Americans more than two hundred years ago, this herb is the most popular botanical in the United States for relieving menopausal symptoms. According to the University of Maryland Medical Center, it has been embraced as a "safe and effective treatment for women who cannot or will not take hormonal replacement therapy for menopause."

Black cohosh's best known hormone-balancing trait, as reported in many scientific journals, is that it contains estrogen-like natural chemicals. The herb can therefore help boost the hormone when you're in menopausal decline.

Another amazing trait: black cohosh may help support weight loss. When estrogen levels fall during menopause, the body increases fat cell production to make and access more estrogen. This is one of the reasons we tend to put on weight at menopause. Some research shows that black cohosh may intervene in this process and that women taking the herb during menopause do lose weight.

Black cohosh has been credited with helping digestive issues, promoting nutrient absorption, and ensuring regular waste removal. This means you may have less constipation, bloating, and gas buildup.

Recommended dosage: This herb is part of my Vida Optimal Balance, a menopausal formula available on my website that is designed to help balance female hormones. Take 1 or 2 capsules twice a day.

If you take black cohosh alone, the following dosages have been studied in research: 20 to 80 mg taken twice daily for menopausal symptoms; and 40 mg daily for weakened bones (osteoporosis).

Chasteberry

As the name suggests, chasteberry is an herb once thought to quash sex drive. According to folklore, medieval monks chewed on the leaves of chasteberry trees in order to help them keep their vows of celibacy.

While it's now clear that the herb does not affect libido, it is one of the most important medicinal plant agents for women's health.

Many scientific papers have been published on chasteberry, confirming that it has anti-inflammatory, antioxidant, anti-diabetic, anti-cancer, and antimicrobial properties.

Chasteberry is also an important herb for weight loss and hormone balance. It stimulates the making of progesterone, which can help to balance out the lack of estrogen during menopause and ease PMS symptoms prior to menopause. Restoring balance improves satiety and increases energy—two benefits that make it easier to stick to your weight-loss plan.

Recommended dosage: This herb is also part of Vida Optimal Balance. Take 1 or 2 capsules twice a day.

If you take chasteberry alone, suggested dosages of the extract (capsules) range from 20 to 40 mg a day, according to clinical trials. Some companies sell 300 mg capsules, which are to be taken once a day. Fluid extract (40 drops daily in the morning) and tincture (35 to 45 drops three times daily) also have been used. Talk to your healthcare practitioner about dosage.

Green Tea

If you want to sip your way to a slimmer body, drink green tea. It is an extraordinary beverage, packed with antioxidants. It also revs up the liver's detoxification system that rids the body of chemicals, toxins, and free radicals that damage cells.

Two of the most powerful compounds in green tea are caffeine and natural chemicals called catechins. Together, they boost metabolism and stimulate weight loss.

Sipping green tea daily, or taking green tea extract, may help you reduce visceral fat too. When overweight people drank a beverage providing 886 mg of catechins and 198 mg of caffeine daily for ninety days, they had the greatest percent decrease in visceral fat, total fat mass, and total body mass, compared to another group who consumed less of the active substances.

Recommended dosage: I advise having two or three cups a day of green tea. Let a tea bag or two steep in hot water for three minutes in order to extract maximum amounts of antioxidants, caffeine, and catechins. Another way to obtain catechins is by supplementing with Vida Optimal Balance and Mighty Maca Plus. Both contain green tea extract.

Maca

This superfood is made from a radish-like tuber that grows above eleven thousand feet in Peru's central highlands. Maca is an adaptogen, which means it can help support your adrenals, especially against the impact of burnout and chronic stress. Maca is beneficial in triggering weight loss. It helps control blood sugar levels in the body, boosts energy for workouts, and regulates hormones—all factors involved in weight control.

Additionally, maca helps keep the body from being too acidic because it is very alkalinizing. Maca also supports hormone balance, sex drive, and mood, and it decreases hot flashes.

Highly nutritious, it is the base of my hormone-balancing supplement Mighty Maca Plus, which also contains other superfoods from around the world, such as turmeric, resveratrol, quercetin, the herb cat's claw, cinnamon, green tea extract, apple fiber, spirulina, and others. These have a potent combined antioxidant effect.

I created Mighty Maca Plus from my journey around the world looking for answers to my health crisis.

I have more than ten years of clinical results and client testimonials praising the benefits clients have gotten with this combination of ingredients, from improvements in blood-sugar control to a reduction in hot flashes, reduced cravings, improvement in aches and pains, better mood, increased libido, and more.

Recommended dosage: One or two scoops daily of Mighty Maca Plus in smoothies, water, or tea is a good way to harness all the powers of this amazing herb.

Maca is also available commercially in several dosage forms besides powder: liquid, tablets, and capsules. These should be taken with food following the formulator's guidelines.

Hormonal Supplements

DHEA

Available as a nutritional supplement or as a topical cream, DHEA is a natural hormone produced by the adrenal glands and ovaries that is converted to estrogen and testosterone. DHEA dwindles dramatically as you age, along with declining insulin efficiency. In postmenopausal women, for example, the production of DHEA is near zero.

Supplementing with DHEA may help with hormone balancing, memory, mood, immune function, muscle development, bone health, and fat-burning. And we know from the study on DHEA that I mentioned in Chapter 1 that DHEA supplements can be belly fat burners.

Recommended dosage: Before supplementing with oral or topical DHEA, have your levels tested. If your DHEA-S (not DHEA) level is low (under 120 µg/dL), I recommend beginning treatment with 5 mg of DHEA per day and slowly working up to what feels like an optimal level. While doses of 10 mg to a crazy 500 mg have been reported, a common dose is 25 to 50 mg per day for men and 5 to 15 mg for women. Your physician should be able to help you adjust your dosage accordingly. The topical vulvar rejuvenating cream I created for women, called Julva, contains approximately 8 mg DHEA per ½ mL (a pea-size amount), in addition to its other rejuvenating ingredients. It has worked very well for dryness and libido!

Melatonin

This hormone is secreted naturally by the tiny pineal gland, located in your brain. It helps regulate your sleep-wake cycle, otherwise known as the circadian rhythm. Adequate levels of melatonin are necessary to fall asleep quickly and sleep soundly through the night.

Although best known as a sleep remedy, melatonin has many other benefits in the body, including weight control. Quite a bit of research has confirmed that a melatonin deficiency correlates with obesity, and that supplementing with melatonin may support weight loss. In a 2017 study, researchers gave thirty obese patients a daily dose of either 10 mg of melatonin or a placebo for thirty days. The patients also followed a calorie-controlled diet.

At the end of the experimental period, only the melatonin group had lost a significant amount of weight. Based on looking at the patients' lab work (before and after the study), the researchers noted that two weight-control hormones, leptin (the "I'm full" hormone) and adiponectin (a major fat-burning hormone), were elevated in the melatonin group. From the results, it appears that melatonin works by enhancing the secretion of these hormones. The researchers concluded that "melatonin should be considered in obesity management." The study was published in *Oxidative Medicine and Cellular Longevity*.

Even if you're not obese or overweight, I recommend supplementing with melatonin if for no other reason than to help ensure you get a good night's sleep.

Recommended dosage: Take 3 mg in the evening, prior to bedtime.

Progesterone (Topical)

If you're over age fifty or if you're struggling with PMS or menstrual irregularities past age forty, I recommend that you consider topical bioidentical progesterone cream. But definitely discuss this treatment with your physician.

Clinical studies continually demonstrate the effectiveness of bioidentical progesterone for hormone balance, bone strength, mood, heart health, better sleep, symptom relief for menopause, and much more. As I mentioned too, age-related declines in progesterone can lead to belly fat, so supplementing with bioidentical progesterone may help you maintain a trim waistline.

Progesterone protects the brain and its interactions, which is why I also recommend topical progesterone to women who have had hysterectomies and no longer produce this hormone. After using bioidentical progesterone, many women have told me, "I feel like a fog has lifted."

My preference is topical progesterone cream formulated with the natural version of the hormone. Why is this important? Most pharmaceutical products actually contain synthetic versions of progesterone called progestins. Far more powerful than the body's own natural progesterone, progestins can be metabolized into toxic by-products that may interfere with your own natural progesterone. This leads to hormone-related health problems and increases the risk of breast cancer in users.

Natural progesterone, on the other hand, is identical to the progesterone produced by your body. It is produced in scientific laboratories from wild yams and soybeans (note, however, that natural progesterone should not be confused with wild yam extracts).

My Pura Balance PPR Cream is a formulation of natural, bioavailable progesterone and pregnenolone, the "mother of all hormones." Pregnenolone levels, like many health-promoting hormones, drop with age. It is an important hormone for many aspects of health and aging well, including bone and brain health.

Recommended dosage: Apply one pump of Pura Balance PPR Cream in the evening to soft skin areas of your body (face, neck, chest, inner arms, and lower abdomen). Massage well into skin. (If you're still having a menstrual cycle, use the cream on days 14 to 28. When post-menopausal, use on days 1 to 25 monthly.)

Other topical over-the-counter progesterone creams typically call for the use of one pump daily as well. With the help of your doctor, prescriptions can be customized for oral forms, troches, or topical application.

Digestive Support Supplements

Digestive Enzymes

At times your food may not be digested fully as it passes through the digestive tract, in which case the nutrients in food are not sufficiently liberated. One main reason for this is a decline in our naturally occurring digestive enzymes as we age.

Normally these enzymes break down food so we can soak up nutrients. When our natural enzyme production falls off, however, we might experience occasional gas, bloating, or indigestion. Supplementation with digestive enzymes can be an effective solution. They help prevent these symptoms, regulate the bowels, and speed detoxification.

Digestive enzymes are formulated with many different types of enzymes. Some of the most common are plant-sourced enzymes like bromelain (from pineapple) and papain (from papaya). They provide proteolytic enzymes that break down proteins. Bromelain and papain also help soothe chronic inflammation in the body.

Other digestive enzymes are sourced from microbes (fungi, yeast, and bacteria). They include amylase, which breaks down starches; protease, which digests gluten and casein (a protein in dairy foods); and lipase, essential for digesting fat.

Digestive formulas can be very useful to take every day with food, usually as an after-meal supplement to encourage the completion of the digestive process. One study reported that people who took enzyme supplements containing lipase, protease, and amylase before and after a fatty meal had fewer digestive problems like gas, bloating, and uncomfortable fullness than the control group. The Keto-Green 16 diet is purposely high in good fats to support ketosis, so digestive enzyme supplements are a perfect companion to the plan.

Recommended dosage: A specific supplement I often recommend is Vida Enzymes. Take 2 capsules with dinner.

There are many different types of digestive enzyme supplements on the market. Follow the manufacturer's recommendation for dosage.

Fiber Complex

Fiber is a big player in weight loss. It contributes to satiety, as well as helping to usher excess calories out of the body. It also helps detoxify the body and provides prebiotics (foods that feed probiotics in the gut).

Fiber supplements are formulated with many different types of ingredients, including beet fiber, psyllium, grain fibers, gums, fructans (which are prebiotics), beta-glucan, and others.

How well fiber supplements work to help with weight loss depends on the type of fiber in the formulation. In a 2017 study published in *Nutrition,* for example, beta-glucan was found to significantly reduce belly fat (by over an inch) after six weeks of use, compared to a placebo group (which actually gained a half-inch on average). Psyllium is another fiber that has been found to trim belly fat.

Recommended dosage: Follow the manufacturer's recommendations. Also, if you're supplementing with my Mighty Maca Plus, it contains a fiber called beta-glucan and other fibers.

Probiotics

I encourage women (and men) to supplement with probiotics, friendly bacteria that empower a healthy gastrointestinal tract. These supplements play a role in weight control too, particularly in trimming belly fat. For one thing, they help detoxify xenoestrogens, unnatural hormones we absorb from our environment. These toxic hormones interfere with weight loss. Second, probiotics support weight loss. A 2014 study published in the *British Journal of Nutrition* revealed that a probiotic supplement helped obese women shed pounds and keep them off. Probiotics further benefit you by curbing the growth of harmful gut bacteria, promoting good digestion, boosting immune function, and increasing your resistance to infection.

Recommended dosage: Take one dose of 30 billion CFUs (colony-forming units) prior to bedtime. Make sure you choose the right formulation. I recommend that you select a probiotic formulated with four of the most highly researched species: *Bifidobacterium lactis, Bifidobacterium longum, Lactobacillus acidophilus,* and *Lactobacillus plantarum.*

A precaution: Do not supplement with probiotics if you have been diagnosed with small intestinal bowel overgrowth (SIBO). Probiotics can aggravate this condition.

Other Key Supplements

Adrenal Glandulars

These extracts are formulated with actual adrenal gland tissue usually derived from bovine (beef) sources. They help human adrenal glands repair themselves so they can heal and function normally again. Thus, an adrenal glandular can be a good source of adrenal support.

Recommended dosage: Follow the manufacturer's recommendation for dosage.

Carnitine

This is an amino acid produced by your body. You can also get it from eating meat or taking it as a supplement. A great deal of proof finds that carnitine can help with weight loss. In a 2016 issue of *Obesity Reviews*, researchers did a systematic review of studies that examined the effect of carnitine on weight loss in adults. The news was good: The subjects who took carnitine lost significantly more weight, without losing muscle, compared with control groups.

Although discovered as a component of the human body over a hundred years ago, carnitine remained virtually unstudied until the last twenty years. Today we know that it is vital to normal body functions, because it transports fatty acids into the mitochondria of cells to be converted to energy. It also removes waste products given off by the mitochondria during energy production. Without carnitine, one of the body's most important "fuel pumps" for energy is cut off.

Recommended dosage: Take 1,000 to 3,000 mg in divided doses — half in the morning and the other half in the evening — each day.

Omega-3 Fish Oil

The important components of fish oil are the omega-3 fatty acids, EPA and DHA. Both can actually reduce body fat—particularly in the belly. Researchers in China did a statistical analysis of seven studies involving omega-3 fats and overweight adults and concluded that supplementation produced a significant reduction in waist circumference. The study was published in 2017 in the *Journal of Nutrition, Health, and Aging*.

Recommended dosage: I advise supplementing with 1,000 mg (including 360 mg EPA and 240 mg DHA) taken once in the morning. It's important to choose a high-quality fish oil that is certified by the International Fish Oils Standards (IFOS), guaranteeing quality, potency, and purity.

BPC-157

New to the market, BPC-157 stands for Body Protein Compound 157. It's a sequence of fifteen amino acids that are linked together to form what is termed a "peptide." BPC-157 is derived from a protective protein found in the stomach of humans and mammals.

After studying BPC-157 research (mostly on lab animals), I was intrigued. This supplement is capable of acting as a brain booster, a performance enhancer, a bone-and-soft-tissue healer, and a remedy for ulcers and problems in the gastrointestinal tract. These are conditions that often plague women in menopause and afterward. One way in which BPC-157 works is through its ability to help the body form new blood vessels, which can then carry healing substances to injured or ill areas of the body.

Recommended dosage: BPC-157 is available as an oral supplement. I advise taking 500 mg daily. (It is not vegan friendly, however.)

Final Tips

Always check with your doctor before taking any supplements, especially if you are on any prescription medications. Look for an expiration date on your supplements, and don't use them past that date. Store them in a cool, dry place.

You can find a number of these supplements on my website dranna.com. Here's an overview:

SUPPLEMENT	PURPOSE	DOSAGE
Pura D3K2	Supports bone health, cardiovascular health, and normal blood clotting.	Take 1 capsule daily.
Vida Optimal Balance	Supports balance of female hormones, may ease symptoms associated with PMS and menopause; promotes estrogen detoxification; and provides antioxidant activity and cellular support.	Take 2 capsules twice daily.
Mighty Maca Plus	Increases stamina and energy; aids metabolism; improves digestion; supports alkalinity; and improves symptoms of hormone imbalance.	1 to 2 scoops daily, mixed in water, bone broth, or smoothies.
Keto-Green Meal Replacement	Provides a meal replacement in the Keto-Green 16 diet.	1 to 2 scoops daily in a smoothie.
Pura Balance PPR cream	Supports bone health, hormone balance, mood, stress relief, and youthful skin.	Apply 1 pump of cream in the evening to soft skin areas of your body (face, neck, chest, inner arms, and lower abdomen). Massage well into skin. If you are still having periods, use on days 14 to 28 each month. If you are menopausal, use on days 1 to 25 each month.
Vida Enzymes	Digestive enzymes to support healthy digestion; break down fats, protein, carbohydrates, fiber, and lactose; and enhance nutrient absorption.	Take 2 capsules with dinner.

(continued)

SUPPLEMENT	PURPOSE	DOSAGE
Pura Probio Max Daily	Helps maintain a healthy gut microbiome, supports immunity, enhances bowel regularity, and supports lactose digestion.	Take 1 capsule daily.
Pura Omega Extreme	Helps prevent inflammation, supports cardiovascular health, enhances brain health, and supports healthy glucose and insulin metabolism.	Take 1 softgel daily.

When selecting a brand of supplements, look for emblems indicating that the product is produced according to GMP and NSF standards. These certifications tell you that the product is a quality one and contains what the label says it contains.

For the most part, take your supplements with meals for optimal absorption. Some of the supplements I've recommended are designed to be taken in divided dosages, which is beneficial because they provide your body with a steady supply of nutrients all day long.

Chapter 8

Not for Women Only: Get Your Man on This Plan!

. . . .

Throughout this book, I've been focusing on the impact of Keto Green nutrition and supplementation on women. But maybe you're asking whether Keto-Green 16 can work for the man (or men) in your life. This is an important question because nearly 75 percent of American men are now obese or overweight (compared to 60 percent of U.S. women), according to the Institute for Health Metrics and Evaluation. Unfortunately, if nothing changes, we're going to see even more obesity and obesity-related health problems among our beloved guys.

Back to your question. The answer is yes, Keto-Green 16 works for men. The shape a man is in, like the shape you're in, has to do with hormones. Because this diet works on balancing weight-control hormones, it boosts weight loss, promotes ketosis, and beats hormone havoc in men too.

I've emphasized that natural hormone decline in women is one of the culprits in weight gain and belly fat and results in a lot of symptoms that affect quality of life and disease progression, especially in and around menopause. Well, a similar transition is happening in men!

As they age, men must navigate through "andropause," in which

they too experience hormonal changes. Andropause is a true condition. Author Gail Sheehy calls it the "unspeakable passage" because
men are reluctant to talk about it. But it is a process that begins during a man's forties or fifties and chips away relentlessly at his
strength, sexuality, outlook on life, and masculinity. Andropause
also causes a man to gain weight, especially around his middle.

Shifting Male Hormones

A man's testosterone peaks in his twenties and gradually declines
about 1 percent a year after the age of thirty. According to the Urology Care Foundation, approximately 20 percent of men in their
sixties have low testosterone (low T), a figure that increases to 30
percent among men in their seventies. I suspect that this number is
higher, however. What is considered "normal" for a man's age does
not necessarily mean "optimal."

Testosterone is a sex hormone important to both men and
women, even though many of you likely think it is only a "guy
thing." In men, testosterone is primarily made by the testicles. In
both men and women, it is produced in much smaller amounts by
the adrenal glands, and in women, it is manufactured by the ovaries.

Testosterone gives a guy increased energy levels, higher self-
esteem, strength and physical stamina, a healthy metabolism, better
bone density, and strength by aiding in the production of red blood
cells in the bone marrow. Testosterone is also essential to prostate
health, liver function, memory, and concentration.

In puberty, testosterone causes a young man to build muscles,
grow facial and body hair, develop a deeper voice, and produce
sperm. In men, testosterone is also important to achieving an erection and plays a clear role in kindling sexual desire, as it does in
women as well.

Testosterone exists in the body in two forms. There's free testosterone, which isn't bound to proteins in the body. This is the form
of testosterone most available to act within the body. It is responsible for male characteristics, sex drive, and muscularity.

Bound testosterone is attached to a protein called sex hormone-binding globulin (SHBG) and isn't active. In other words, SHBG keeps some of the testosterone captive, so it can't do much. If tests show you have a high level of SHBG, this means that it is likely that less free testosterone is available to your tissues. A low SHBG level means that more of the testosterone is free, bioavailable, and not bound to SHBG.

Total testosterone is a measure of how much testosterone you have in your blood in total, both free and bound.

According to the American Association for Clinical Chemistry (AACC), free testosterone only accounts for 1 to 4 percent of the testosterone in a typical male's bloodstream. Your doctor can get measures of both types of testosterone and other hormones, using a simple blood test.

Testing for Low Testosterone

A diagnosis of low testosterone is typically made if a man's free testosterone hormone level is below 300 ng/dL. As a physician specializing in hormonal and sexual health, I typically consider optimal male testosterone levels to be somewhere between 600 to 900 ng/dL—rarely above or below those numbers. The tests that I routinely recommend to my male clients include biomarkers: testosterone (free and total), SHBG, estradiol, total estrogen, cortisol, DHEA-S, thyroid-stimulating hormone (TSH), free T3, free T4, thyroid antibodies, hemoglobin A1c (HbA1c), vitamin D, hsCRP, and homocysteine.

Testing is the only way you can validate a low-T diagnosis and measure treatment progress. Your doctor may suspect you have hormone imbalances by your symptoms, but you should ask for testing to confirm unhealthy levels. Testing also ensures your doctor rules out other issues that may simply have similar symptoms. With your test results in hand, your physician can best determine what the optimal levels are for you and determine the best course of treatment.

Low T and Male Health

Although a gradual decline in testosterone levels is part of the normal aging process in men, it has a negative impact on the body. Low testosterone levels increase body fat, especially around the middle, and reduce muscle mass. A typical American male can lose twelve to twenty pounds of muscle between the ages of forty and seventy. He may also lose 15 percent of his bone mass and nearly two inches in height.

If a man becomes obese, a vicious cycle ensues. An obese man is more likely to have low testosterone. And a man with low testosterone is more likely to get obese.

As a man's free testosterone declines, he may start to experience a wide variety of other symptoms and health concerns:

- Brain fog and fatigue

- Depression

- Night sweats (testosterone is important to a good night's sleep)

- Mood swings

- Increase in abdominal fat (testosterone inhibits fat accumulation)

- Elevated cholesterol

- Anxiety and irritability

- Increased risk of insulin resistance and diabetes

- Osteopenia/osteoporosis (testosterone improves bone density)

- Decreased stamina

- Decreased muscle mass (testosterone helps maintain lean muscle mass)

- Decreased mental ability (testosterone synthesizes neurotransmitters, so improves brain function)

- Decreased erection (testosterone is essential for libido, arousal, and orgasm)

- Decreased urine flow

- Greater risk of heart disease

Does anyone think these look a lot like the key symptoms seen in menopause?

WHAT PORN DOES TO A MAN'S TESTOSTERONE LEVELS

Porn. The very word is enough to grab attention. Now that I've got yours, let me start out by saying that research shows that in men with low testosterone levels and those with erectile dysfunction (ED), the actual act of sex is better than watching porn for increasing testosterone naturally. What's more, masturbation combined with porn torpedoes testosterone levels, leaving a guy drained, unmotivated, and often filled with shame and guilt.

Surprised? I'm sure you are. Looking at porn is not a good idea in general, and especially if a man is testosterone challenged or is having sexual dysfunction issues.

Kinsey Institute researchers were among the first to report pornography-induced erectile dysfunction and pornography-induced abnormally low libido, in 2007. Men were recruited from bars and bathhouses, where video pornography was everywhere. They were unable to achieve erections in the lab in response to video porn.

Many other clinicians have also described pornography-related sexual dysfunctions. For example, in his book *The*

New Naked, urology professor Harry Fisch reported that excessive Internet pornography use impaired sexual performance in his patients, and psychiatry professor Norman Doidge reported in his book *The Brain That Changes Itself* that removal of Internet pornography use reversed impotence and sexual arousal problems in his patients.

Surprisingly, the average male has 22 percent less testosterone now than in 1980 (which was when scientists first measured levels in the United States). Why is this? The big reason is lifestyle. People eat bad food. They exercise less. And there's more technology—namely, the Internet. Men watch pornography more today, especially online, than ever before.

I look at pornography from a medical perspective, having treated many men and women to help them improve their sex lives. My hope here is that people of *both* sexes who read this section will take from it a compassionate stance. However, if you or someone you love has been struggling with a pornography habit or experiencing sexual problems, it is time to take an honest look at your relationship with pornography and realize that it may be eroding your sexuality, testosterone, and masculinity—and, most importantly, your intimate relationships.

Enter Estrogen

A man's level of testosterone is only part of the equation. Another hormone is involved—estrogen. Yes, men have estrogen just like women. In fact, the average sixty-year-old man has more circulating estrogen in his blood than the average sixty-year-old woman. Let that sink in!

Where is all this estrogen coming from?

There are many factors that contribute to an increase in estrogen in men as they age. One factor is likely the result of increased exposure to hormone disruptors in the environment, many of which mimic estrogen and are feminizing to men. Hormone disruptors are found in processed food, the environment, household cleaners, plastics, sunscreens, and personal care products.

Not only do hormone disruptors increase estrogen, but they are also responsible for dwindling total testosterone levels in men. So reducing exposure to these can help restore hormone balance. Switching to chemical-free, organic products can help. So can avoiding plastics and avoiding drinking liquids from plastic containers.

Another factor is that estrogen is found in our food, especially non-organic meats and dairy. This is why I advise everyone to eat grass-fed beef and other organic proteins because they do not contain the hormones given to conventionally grown cows and chickens. As for seafood, look for wild-caught fish. Choices like these lift the burden of exposure to harmful estrogens in the environment.

The final and most significant factor is the activity of certain enzymes in the body, called aromatase enzymes. Found in fat tissue, the brain, the testes, blood vessels, and skin, these enzymes convert testosterone into the normal small amounts of estrogen needed for bones, skeletal strength, and other processes in men.

But as men age, aromatase enzyme activity falls off. This is where the problem occurs. More and more of the already diminishing testosterone is converted to more and more estrogen. This results in all of the typical low T symptoms but also impacts a man's underlying health, partly due to the increase in estrogen. One distressing problem with too much estrogen is that hormone acts like a fat magnet, locking it in around a man's middle. Getting off sugar and processed foods helps prevent declines in aromatase enzymes.

Research has shown that high estrogen raises diabetes risk and increases the risk for prostate cancer and autoimmune diseases. There are conflicting views on whether low T and/or high estrogen increases heart disease in men, but my dear friend Dr. Steven Masley, author of several books on heart health, wrote an article about a study that focused on the health benefits of increasing testosterone to healthy levels. When men with low T (less than 300 ng/dL) had their testosterone levels restored to normal levels (500–1,000 ng/dL), they experienced the following results:

- 47 percent decrease in risk of death

- 18 percent reduction in heart attacks

- 30 percent decrease in risk of stroke

This is proof positive that declining testosterone levels are not ordained; they can be revived, and it's not too late.

Hormone Restoration in Men

I have worked with many men over the course of my medical career to bring them back in hormonal balance, normal weight, and better health. One of the best examples is my father. My dad was in my life for an amazing fifty years, until he passed away at age ninety-one. But we almost lost him twelve years earlier.

Dad, a U.S. Navy veteran who fought in World War II, suffered from diabetes and was in generally poor health and severely overweight. As far as his doctor was concerned, at age seventy-nine my father was a "lost cause," and the doctor thought we shouldn't expect too much more of him. But I knew that my dad had a long life ahead of him, and my dad knew it too.

I was convinced that his chief issue was one of diet, lifestyle, and hormones, and my father agreed to let me take charge of making changes in those departments. I helped him upgrade his diet, gave him supplements and testosterone injections, and slowly and gradually weaned him off three prescription medicines.

As for his weight, Dad lost thirty pounds in thirty days by following an earlier version of my Keto-Green diet. He was able to decrease his daily insulin usage from 120 units to 20 units. Plus he went from being so easily fatigued that he often needed a wheelchair to getting out on the tennis court again.

As a result of taking care of his health, my father was able to return to his home in Pennsylvania and live on his own—driving, shopping, traveling, and loving life! When he turned eighty-nine, however, the long-standing complications of diabetes took their toll on his kidneys. He ended up in the ICU with kidney failure and was put on dialysis. According to statistics, when someone over age seventy is put on dialysis, the average life expectancy is six months. But Dad lived two more years—to ninety-one!

My experience with my father taught me a lot: It's not too late to turn someone's health around and put more life into those years. You too can make a new man out of your husband, boyfriend, son, father, or best friend by following my Keto-Green principles. Never give up! Here's how.

The Keto-Green 16 Diet and Lifestyle for Men

Start with Keto-Green

The first and most important move a man should make to rebalance his hormones is to lose weight. Remember, overweight or obesity makes a man's testosterone plummet. Losing weight helps correct it, not to mention that it makes a guy feel better about himself—more virile, fit, and energetic.

My clinical research shows that this diet works for men of all ages. Case in point: Timothy decided to go Keto-Green for sixteen days because he wanted to lose weight. He lost ten pounds in that period, dropping from 209.8 to 199.8 pounds, and most of the loss was fat because he trimmed an inch off his middle (41 inches to 40 inches) in no time at all. Timothy told me, "It was as if I was melting fat from my stomach like butter." Further, he felt good on the diet, with minimal keto flu symptoms, and he enjoyed the food choices.

Another success story is Chris, who was fifty pounds overweight. "I didn't like how I looked, and I certainly didn't like how

I felt. I had no energy and no motivation in my life," he told me. "I was just a fat dad on the couch watching TV after dinner every day and trying not to fall asleep at 7 P.M."

Chris started the Keto-Green 16 plan and easily dropped a pound a day. Because he had more weight to lose, he continued eating the Keto-Green way. The weight continued falling off, and he had the energy to resume an exercise program. "Now I'm very fit, in fact. I'm running a Spartan Sprint [an extreme obstacle course 5K race] in just a few days, and I'm signed up for a second one in a few months. I have all kinds of dreams and goals, and I'm literally chasing after them because I have the energy and the focus I haven't had in years."

And he no longer craves unhealthy junk food. "When I see things I shouldn't eat, it doesn't even register in my brain. It's like what a non-smoker feels like when they see a pack of cigarettes—they have nothing to do with them, so they don't even notice them."

Chris describes his life as "aging in reverse." "Before, I was like an old man with no get-up-and-go, and now I feel unstoppable. I used to struggle with strange symptoms, like random aches and pains and skin problems, but all that has disappeared now that my hormones have balanced."

Men can really tackle their weight with this diet. It's effective for male hormonal balance, diabetes, heart disease, and energy. Let me add that it's great for a man's libido and sexual function. In my studies, the men reported less sexual dysfunction across the board.

The Keto-Green 16 diet emphasizes whole foods full of good healthy fats, adequate protein, lots of alkalinizing veggies like greens, and very few carbohydrates. With fewer carbs to use for fuel, the body relies on fat.

The plan is also high in B vitamins, folate, choline, and betaine—helpful in supporting methylation, a process in the body that helps metabolize and detoxify excess estrogens that may have built up in a man's body. Fish and spinach are particularly high in these methylators.

Also important for decreasing estrogen are the cruciferous veggies on the plan, such as broccoli, cabbage, cauliflower, and Brussels sprouts. They are loaded with glucosinolates, which help scale back harmful estrogen activity, along with reducing weight so that body fat doesn't store estrogens.

Men do extremely well on low-carbohydrate diets like this one. Plus, they can eat a little more dietary fat and protein than a woman is allowed. Fat is filling and energizing—which makes it easy for a guy to stick with the food plan.

So get your guy to follow the Keto-Green 16 diet with you!

THE DARK SIDE OF BLUE LIGHT

Blue light wavelengths, which are emitted by electronic screens, seem to be the most disruptive at night. They trigger your body to produce more daytime hormones, such as cortisol. When cortisol goes up, your testosterone goes down. So does levels of the sleep hormone, melatonin—which means you don't sleep as well. Since your body produces a majority of its testosterone while you sleep, you're killing tomorrow's testosterone levels if you're tossing and turning.

So I recommend using blue-light shielding glasses or electronic covers when you're in front of computer screens for long periods of time, or shutting down your electronics at least a few hours before bed to protect testosterone production.

Supplements for Hormonal Support

I've reversed andropause symptoms such as erectile dysfunction, low libido, weight gain, and fatigue in men through natural means, without prescription medications, in many cases. Once your guy is on the diet 100 percent, I suggest adding in the following supplements.

Multivitamin/mineral

Start here to create a solid nutritional support foundation. Men with nutrient deficiencies are at a hormonal and health disadvantage, increasing the risk for bone weakness, loss of muscle, poor mood, and low energy.

I recommend a multivitamin/mineral blend featuring activated vitamins, including folate as 5-MTHF (5-methyltetrahydrofolate), and Albion chelated mineral complexes because these are well absorbed.

Recommended dosage: If the formulation is meant to be taken in divided doses, take 2 capsules daily—one in the morning or at lunch, and one in the evening. Alternatively, take a once-a-day multivitamin/mineral supplement.

Zinc

Many men, especially over the age of sixty, have low zinc levels. This shortfall correlates with low testosterone and low semen output, which is why this mineral is so important to hormone balance. Zinc provides global protection in other areas—fertility, immunity, and insulin sensitivity, to name just a few, as well as dopamine production, which helps support mood, sex drive, and zest for life.

Recommended dosage: I typically recommend 50 to 60 mg per day. I suggest protein-rich foods and fermented foods such as sauerkraut and kimchi. It's a good idea for men to substitute oysters for fish on the Keto-Green 16 plan, since oysters are the richest source of zinc on the planet.

Vitamin D

This nutrient is actually technically a hormone, not a vitamin, and is important for both men and women. A simple blood test can measure levels.

I like to see clients maintain a serum blood level between 50 and 80 ng/mL. Studies have shown that men with lower levels of vitamin D have lower levels of testosterone.

Vitamin D3 supplements are widely available (best is to get one that contains vitamin K as well, as that allows for better absorption of the vitamin D), and you can also bump up your sunlight exposure.

Recommended dosage: If a man tests below my preferred range, I typically recommend 5,000 IU a day, until the levels improve, of one like my vitamin D/K2 supplement, available at dranna.com.

DHEA

For men, supplementation with DHEA has been found to:

- Reduce bone and muscle loss

- Address and improve thinning skin

- Reduce body fat

- Prevent type 2 diabetes

- Boost memory and cognition

- Improve sexual desire, arousal, and orgasm

Recommended dosage: Generally, I recommend 25–50 mg for men, depending on tested levels (levels need to be tested and monitored by a physician).

Adrenal Support

Stress generates too much fat-forming cortisol and shuts down sexual hormones (such as testosterone) as our bodies go into fight-or-flight mode. Supplements called adaptogens, which nourish the adrenals, are key to correcting those imbalances.

One of the best adaptogens is a powder that I sell on my website, Mighty Maca Plus. Maca supports hormone balance, sex drive, and mood. What's more, it has been clinically proven to improve erection, sperm production, and sperm motility.

Additionally, maca helps keep the body from being too acidic (stress is extremely acidifying by itself) because it is very alkalinizing.

Maca comes in powdered form, as a liquid, and in capsules.

Recommended dosage: If you're using my Mighty Maca Plus, have 2 scoops daily in water or as part of a Keto-Green smoothie. Other helpful additions are vitamin C (a daily dose of 500 to 2,000 mg, taken any time of the day), carnitine (2,000 to 6,000 mg daily), and an omega-3 fatty acid supplement (1 capsule daily). For omega-3s, I prefer Pura Omega Extreme (see the appendix "Keto-Green 16 Resources") or OmegaPure 600EC from Xymogen.

Testoplex (by Xymogen)

I have recommended this supplement to men for years. It is a special formulation to address healthy testosterone levels and provide support for libido and overall vitality. It features mung bean sprout powder, which addresses healthy testosterone levels and provides support for libido and overall vitality.

Recommended dosage: Take 2 capsules in the morning, or as directed by your healthcare practitioner.

L-arginine

This amino acid may be a natural Viagra. That's because it boosts the production of nitric oxide in the body. Nitric oxide (not to be confused with nitrous oxide, or laughing gas) is a molecule that helps to relax and expand blood vessels (vasodilation). Arginine is the only amino acid that serves as a building block for nitric oxide. Taking supplemental arginine can help the blood vessels in the penis dilate, and you know what that means: firmer erections.

Arginine also can increase growth hormone by blocking the release of growth-hormone-inhibiting hormone. When this chemical, which inhibits the release of the hormone, is blocked, growth hormone levels begin to climb. This effect can be seen about thirty minutes after taking arginine.

Recommended dosage: Take arginine twice a day; base your dosage on the manufacturer's suggestion. I usually recommend a slow-release arginine supplement made with a beetroot powder called Neo40 by Neogenesis or N.O. Max ER by Xymogen.

Liver/Gallbladder Support

If you've had your gallbladder removed, I recommend this type of supplement. A good one is LV/GB Complex by Designs for Health. It supports bile flow for the normal processing and elimination of toxins through the specific combination of nutrients and herbs in this formula, including L-methionine, taurine, beta-carotene, ox bile, B vitamins, and milk thistle.

Recommended dosage: Take 3 capsules daily with meals.

MEET DR. LIFE!

Recently I interviewed the phenomenal Dr. Jeff Life, a family practice physician in Charleston, West Virginia. You've probably seen him: He's that ripped, muscular healthy older guy in the Cenegenics ads in magazines. Yes—that's who I'm talking about!

At one time, though, he was not the muscular picture of health we see in his photographs today. At age fifty-nine, Dr. Life was overweight, and poorly conditioned, with rapidly declining health.

Determined to reverse his failing health, he began by eating a low-sugar diet, taking supplements, and plunging into an intense strength training routine. By the time he was sixty, after consistently eating right and training hard, he became the grand champion in Bill Phillip's 1998 Body-for-Life contest.

In 2012, *Men's Fitness* selected Dr. Life as one of the top twenty-five fittest men in America. The other twenty-four honorees were men in their twenties and thirties, and most were professional athletes or actors. Today Dr. Life is eighty and still in superb health and condition.

To help other men, he shared with me his top twelve biohacks for men (women can use these too) to stay young and healthy for life:

1. Keep your blood sugar low. (As I do, he recommends the Freestyle Libre glucose monitoring system.)

2. Exercise daily—cardio, flexibility, and strength work. (A flexible man is a sexual man.)

3. Maintain your muscle mass and strength.

4. Avoid and eliminate belly fat.

5. Maintain optimal hormone levels.

6. Maintain ideal blood pressure (below 120/80).

7. Minimize arterial inflammation (diet is important here).

8. Take essential supplements.

9. Lead a purposeful life.

10. Achieve great sleep.

11. Build great relationships with family and friends.

12. Protect your arteries. (Note: If you have erectile dysfunction, this is a precursor to cardiovascular disease. Don't be in denial; see your physician immediately.)

Sexual health for men and women is lifelong and enhances intimacy. I so believe in unlocking our sexual energy to enhance our marriage and our relationship with ourselves that I created an entire course at SexualCPR.com. My full interview with Dr. Life is part of that program. I consider this course required viewing for all women—and men too!

Look into Bioidentical Hormone Replacement

Over the years, I have successfully treated many men with low T. My treatment of choice often includes a combination of bioidentical hormones. These are made from natural compounds and are identical to our body's own natural hormones, which means they are more easily metabolized and utilized by the body without the negative side effects often associated with synthetic hormones.

Testosterone hormone replacement therapy can consist of creams, gels, pellets inserted under the skin, injections, and oral tablets. Men need to be cautious with creams and gels because contact with children or partners can result in their absorbing the testosterone.

Some of the benefits of bioidentical testosterone include:

- Better mood and brain function

- Stronger bone health

- Increased muscle

- Reduced prostate size and overall improvement in prostate health, including a lower PSA and less urgency to urinate during the night

- Improved sexual function and erections

Men may also do well with 5 to 10 mg of a topical progesterone cream at bedtime because it can help trim body fat around the middle. Too little progesterone in men contributes to belly fat. But a little goes a long way; a man should use it only under his doctor's supervision. An option is a half pump of my Pura Balance PPr Cream at bedtime.

ARE THESE MEDS MAKING YOU FAT OR MESSING WITH YOUR WEIGHT AND SEX DRIVE?

Have your doctor review your medications. Some medicines can cause certain people to put on weight. If you are already overweight, weight gain might be more of a problem.

Medication-related weight gain can have many causes. Some drugs might make you very hungry, causing you to eat more and gain extra weight. Others might slow down the metabolism, resulting in the body burning calories at a slower rate. And some medicines might adversely affect how your body stores and absorbs sugars and other nutrients.

Medications that may cause weight gain in men and women include:

- Drugs for diabetes: insulin, thiazolidinediones, and sulfonylureas

- Antipsychotics: haloperidol, clozapine, risperidone, olanzapine, and lithium

- Antidepressants: amitriptyline, imipramine, paroxetine, and sertraline

- Epilepsy medicines: valproate, carbamazepine, and gabapentin

- Steroid hormones like prednisone

- Blood pressure–reducing medicines: propranolol and metoprolol (beta-blockers)

Other medicines may make a guy feel less than frisky by interfering with hormone balance. For example:

- Anti-androgen drugs: flutamide, GNRH analogues, and chemotherapeutic agents

- Psychoactive drugs and mood stabilizers

- Sleeping pills

- Antidepressants

- Blood pressure–reducing medicines

- Others: cimetidine (for peptic ulcer), steroids, aldosterone, lovastatin

- Alcohol (sorry!)

Your physician may be able to prescribe a substitute drug that does not cause weight gain or sexual dysfunction.

As you can see by now, much of how much we weigh, how we feel, how we look, and how we age is rooted in our hormones. The hormone health of both parties in a relationship is vital and should be foremost on a couple's respective minds. Support each other by going Keto-Green together. It can really make a difference in your lives.

Part Three

Live the
Keto-Green 16 Lifestyle

Chapter 9

The 16-Minute Fitness Plan

. . . .

One simple addition to going Keto-Green can help you drop fat pounds, tone your whole body, and trim your belly. The secret is my 16-minute fitness plan, which combines the calorie burning of cardio with the body sculpting of strength training in one very short workout.

Fitness and Your Hormones

This fitness plan is designed not only to firm you up but also to help you take control of your hormones, so that you can burn fat even more efficiently. Hormones are very involved in both building new lean muscle and burning fat, so it's important to have an understanding of which ones are impacted directly by exercise.

Insulin

As we've seen, insulin can cause fat to be stored in the body instead of being used to fuel muscle activity. Fortunately, exercise prevents this kind of fat buildup. It makes muscle cells more receptive to insulin. So when insulin arrives at cells to usher in glucose for energy, the cells welcome them both. This stabilizes your blood sugar and prevents insulin from piling up in the bloodstream and promoting fat storage.

Cortisol

When too high for too long, this stress hormone quickly takes over and brings on food cravings and weight gain. So cortisol levels are something we want to rein in. One important way to do this is by reducing stress, and there's no denying that regular exercise is a great stress reducer.

Oxytocin

Have you ever noticed that you're more affectionate, you're more compassionate, and you feel better about yourself and others when you exercise regularly? These wonderful feelings are all because of the production of oxytocin while you are moving and exercising. Exercise helps activate the release of oxytocin, which in turn energizes us to move even more, in all kinds of healthy and loving ways. Although oxytocin is not an endorphin per se, when oxytocin is released by the pituitary gland, it stimulates the production of endorphins, the "feel-good" hormones most of us have already heard about. The release of more oxytocin also lowers cortisol. (This is probably the reason I am so much happier when I leave the gym!)

Glucagon

The pancreas releases this hormone in response to low blood sugar. Once in circulation, glucagon stimulates the release of fatty acids from fat stores and increases blood glucose levels, both of which help fuel exercise activity. So not only do you burn more fat, you access more energy to exercise harder—which in turn revs up your metabolism.

Growth Hormone

This muscle-building, fat-burning hormone is stimulated by high-intensity exercise such as strength training and cardio workouts. Once released, growth hormone (GH) initiates muscle protein synthesis, or MPS, the process involved in developing nice, firm muscles. If you think of muscle like a brick wall, each brick is a protein. MPS is the addition of new bricks to the wall. GH is like the brick mason who helps build that wall.

Estrogen

Estrogen helps metabolize fat, but it also puts fat where it is supposed to go—like your breasts and hips. When estrogen levels drop off with menopause, your body starts storing fat around the abdominal area, which increases your risk for heart disease. But by building more muscle with exercise, you increase your metabolism, which in turn helps fight fat all over your body.

On the other hand, we're exposed to harmful estrogens in everything from plastics to pesticides in the environment. This can lead to estrogen dominance starting at around age thirty-five. Too much estrogen in the body is a risk factor for breast cancer. Exercise helps lower this risk.

Testosterone

Like growth hormone, testosterone is also responsible for muscle protein synthesis and the repair of muscle damaged by exercise. Therefore, it plays a significant role in helping develop body-firming muscle and attractive curves. Exercise, especially strength training, stimulates the production of testosterone.

The bottom line is that regular exercise is more important than many of us may think, and just moving your body a little each day does wonders for helping balance your hormones. With a regular exercise routine, you may even feel more centered and grounded than you ever have before.

So what's the best exercise to balance these hormones? All exercise is beneficial as long as you enjoy it. Personally, I love to do yoga, walk, do weight training, play tennis or pickleball, and box—and I do one of these practically every day.

Less Is More!

There was a point in my life when I believed that working out for 45 to 60 minutes or longer a day was the best way to lose weight and get fit. But with my crazy schedule as a physician, I found I didn't have time to work out that much, and when I did, I felt draggy and not so great. In fact, I felt old! And I was only in my early forties.

It wasn't until I took up boxing for exercise that I realized that less is more. Boxing workouts typically last no more than 20 or 30 minutes and involve a combo of cardio and strength moves. I was surprised to discover that this shorter workout allowed me to inhabit a body that looks and feels better than ever.

Then I began reading a lot of research showing that shorter bouts of exercise—particularly high-intensity interval training or HIIT (discussed later in this chapter)—are more effective, especially for fat loss and hormone balance. No wonder I was feeling stronger, younger, and healthier!

Australian researchers, for example, found that women who did intervals—they alternated just 8 seconds of high-intensity cardio exercise with 12 seconds of low-intensity, slower activity for 20 minutes three times a week—trimmed down faster than steady-paced exercisers who worked out twice as long. The interval exercisers dropped up to sixteen pounds of fat, shrank their bellies by 12 percent and their thighs by 15 percent, and developed, on average, 1½ pounds of metabolism-revving muscle in fifteen weeks—without dieting.

Something else I learned: Too much exercise is bad for our hormones! For instance, overexercising can really do a number on increasing stress hormones like cortisol, leading to fatigue. It can also increase the risk of muscle loss, increased infections, and injury.

I started hearing from patients and clients that they were busy and couldn't find the time to exercise. With my commitment to shorter workouts deepening, I became determined to create a routine that was fast but that delivered results. It had to provide cardio and sculpting, plus work abs and core. And it had to be short—with no wasted minutes or effort—so that it could fit into anyone's day.

What I landed on was a 16-minute fitness plan based on high-intensity interval training.

HIIT It!

HIIT is a type of short workout that has been shown to burn fat more effectively than regular bouts of steady aerobic exercise. As well as strengthening your lungs and heart, it also increases growth hormone, which tends to decline rapidly as we age. HIIT also improves insulin sensitivity, a great result for your waistline and risk of serious disease. The boxing I do is a form of HIIT.

With HIIT, you can reap the benefits of cardio and strength while maximizing your fat burn in a short amount of time. The "intervals" in HIIT involve alternating between short bursts of hard effort and short periods of less effort.

The alternating intensity resets your metabolism so that it stays high long after you've stopped exercising. This is a phenomenon known as excess post-exercise oxygen consumption (EPOC). It means you burn calories long after you've finished your workout. HIIT accomplishes EPOC better than working out at a continuous moderate pace, according to a 2017 study published in the *European Journal of Applied Physiology*.

HIIT is really powerful during menopause. Falling estrogen causes your metabolism to slow down. The magnitude of that change is that you burn about 50 fewer calories a day. That might not seem like a lot, but it can add up over time if you don't exercise intensely enough—you could put on a pound of fat every twelve weeks.

That fat tends to be of the dangerous kind. Rather than sticking to your hips and thighs, it tends to relocate around your belly, surrounding your organs and increasing the risk of heart disease and diabetes.

Here's where HIIT comes to the rescue: It gets your metabolism back in shape, strengthens your muscles, and burns fat all over, especially around your waistline. Many doctors and fitness professionals are now saying that HIIT may be the perfect exercise for women in menopause.

So if you've got just 16 minutes, you've got time for this killer HIIT workout. It doesn't take hours a day to get in great shape—in only 16 minutes, this workout will deliver fat-burning and muscle-toning benefits.

You might be wondering if you can really get results in 16 minutes. The answer is *yes*. The secret is in the combination of strength moves with cardio moves, done in quick intervals. You're getting a cardio workout for your heart and for torching fat, while sculpting your entire body with resistance exercises that use weights, your body weight, or exercise bands. It is intense, but 16 minutes goes by fast—about the time it takes to do laundry, clean your kitchen after dinner, or wait in line somewhere. Note: For this HIIT workout to genuinely qualify as high-intensity interval training, the effort you put in has to be really intense.

Now let's get sweaty!

The Routine

You can literally do this routine anywhere. I've included moves that target every major muscle group, including the glutes, quads, hamstrings, abs, core, shoulders, and back. Moving through the exercises at a fast pace with little to no rest ensures you'll keep your heart rate elevated, getting a fat-burning cardio effect to boot.

What You'll Need

- Supportive athletic or walking shoes

- A watch with a second hand or timer or smartphone timer

- A resistance band, or two dumbbells that you can lift comfortably for the first several repetitions but then require more effort during the final repetitions

- An exercise mat or a spot on the floor where you can get to work

Quick note about resistance bands: They're versatile and provide enough resistance to make any workout insanely effective. Lightweight and portable, bands are also perfect for traveling or when you're on-the-go.

How to Gauge Your Intensity of Effort

If you have any health conditions or don't exercise regularly, check with your doctor before trying these routines. But if you're cleared to get started, here's what to expect.

During lower-intensity portions of this workout, you'll be doing strength moves with your own body weight or with your resistance band. With these intervals, you should be able to easily carry on a conversation.

When you kick it into high gear with jumping jacks or marching in place, push yourself to the point in which talking is nearly impossible.

Each segment of this workout lasts 1 minute, for a total of sixteen segments and 16 minutes. My general rule of thumb is to just listen to your body. If you find that you feel energized and amazing after a workout, then keep up what you are doing. If you're totally fatigued and feel depleted, it's time to dial things back a bit—reduce the intensity, and go a little more slowly.

Workout Sequence

30 seconds of marching in place to get warmed up

1 minute of jumping jacks, modified jumping jacks, dance with
light jumping, or jumping rope

1 minute of push-ups (chest, arms, shoulders, lower back, and core)

1 minute of marching in place

1 minute of squats (thighs)

1 minute of marching in place

1 minute of biceps curls with a resistance band (biceps)

1 minute of jumping jacks, modified jumping jacks, dance with
light jumping, or jumping rope

1 minute of triceps dips using a chair (triceps)

1 minute of marching in place

1 minute of side lunges (inner thighs and buttocks)

1 minute of jumping jacks, modified jumping jacks, dance with
light jumping, or jumping rope

1 minute of overhead presses with a resistance band (shoulders)

1 minute of marching in place

1 minute of back rows with a resistance band (back)

1 minute of jumping jacks, modified jumping jacks, dance with
light jumping, or jumping rope

1 minute of crunches (abs)

30 seconds of marching slowly in place to cool down

Exercise Instructions

Before you jump into the routine, please read over these instruc-
tions very carefully. Practice each exercise until you have mastered
it. Then you'll be ready to perform the entire workout sequence.

Jumping Jacks
Stand with your feet together and your arms at your sides. Jump
both feet out to the side while raising your arms overhead. Move as
fast as you can. If a regular jumping jack feels hard on your knees,

do a modified jumping jack by stepping out side to side instead of jumping while raising your arms.

Push-ups

On your exercise mat or the floor, get into a high plank, with your palms flat on the mat, arms extended and straight, hands shoulder width apart, and your fingers facing forward.

Slowly lower your body toward the mat, keeping your head aligned with your spine, until your chest or chin is close to the ground. Press back upward with your arms until they are fully extended at your elbows and you're back in the plank, at the top of the push-up position. Repeat the downward and upward movements. If you can't complete a traditional push-up, try doing them with your knees resting on the mat.

Squats

Place your feet a little wider than hip width apart on the floor and point your toes out at a 45-degree angle. Keep your weight in your heels, your back flat, and your chest upright. Bend your knees and lower yourself until your thighs are parallel to the floor. Hold for a moment, then push back to the starting position. Repeat.

Biceps Curls

Stand on the resistance band with your feet placed hip width apart. Grasp a handle in each hand. Alternatively, hold a dumbbell in each hand. Keep your back straight, head straight, chest up, and abs tight. Begin with your arms straight down with your palms facing forward and elbows at your sides. Bend your elbows and pull the handles or dumbbells up to chest height. Lower and repeat.

Triceps Dips

With your fingers pointing forward, place the palms of your hands on a sturdy chair or a low bench, with your back to the chair. Extend your legs straight out in front of you. Bending from your elbows, lower your body as far as you can, then press up to the original position. You should really feel this exercise in the backs of your arms.

Side Lunges

Stand with your feet hip width apart. Keep your body weight in your heels. Step to the left in a deep lateral lunge, keeping your knee above your toes. Come back up to starting position, and do the same to the right. Alternate legs.

Overhead Presses

Stand with one foot slightly in front of the other. Stand on the band with your front foot. Grip a handle in each hand. With the band in front of your arms and palms facing forward, press your arms straight up over your head and together until your arms are almost fully straight. Slowly lower to the starting position and repeat.

You can use dumbbells instead. Grip the weights in each hand. Hold them at shoulder level, elbows bent, and palms facing forward. Press your arms straight up over your head and together until your arms are almost fully straight. Slowly lower to the starting position and repeat.

Back Row

Sit on your mat or floor. Wrap the resistance band under your feet and sit up straight. Grasp the handles in each hand. With your arms extended forward, pull the band back as far as you can toward your abdomen. Hold momentarily as you squeeze your shoulder blades together. Release and extend your arms back out to full extension. Repeat.

To use dumbbells instead of the resistance band, do the following standing exercise: Grasp the dumbbells in each hand. Bend forward slightly, with one foot slightly in front of the other. Bend your elbows and hold the weights close to your sides. Then row upward, squeezing your shoulder blades at the top of the movement. Slowly lower the weights until both arms are fully extended toward the floor. Row back up and repeat.

Crunches

Lie on your mat or on the floor with your feet extended and your elbows bent with your fingers just cupping your head on each side. From this position, lift your upper body up off the floor, using the strength of your abs, until your shoulder blades are off the floor. Then slowly lower yourself down again until your back is once again flat on the floor or mat. Repeat.

Other Hormone-Balancing Moves for Weight Control

Tackling our weight and hormonal issues with exercise is not limited to just HIIT. There are many other activities you can try in order to mix it up and avoid exercise boredom—and still work on getting your hormones back in balance and your body at its happy weight.

Tai Chi

Often described as "meditation in motion," tai chi is an ancient Chinese practice that involves a series of movements performed in a slow, focused manner and accompanied by deep breathing.

A detailed review published in *Worldviews on Evidence-Based Nursing* in 2017 reported that tai chi improved many symptoms related to fluctuating hormones: bodily pain, general health, vitality, mental health, and spinal strength. Many health clubs and gyms offer tai chi classes, which might be worth checking out if you're struggling with symptoms associated with hormonal imbalance.

Walking

Here's a do-anywhere activity that relieves symptoms and builds health. A study of 157 women found that walking with long strides three times a week or more had an awesome impact on PMS symptoms. The women slept better, were less irritable, had fewer joint or muscle pains, were more energetic, and had better sex. They also lost weight, especially around their bellies. The study was published in the journal *Menopause* in 2014.

If you're new to walking, begin your first week by walking just 20 minutes three times a week. The next few weeks, increase your time to 30 minutes. Try to walk a little faster each time. As you feel stronger and more fit, add more walking to your weekly program. Make it your goal to walk five times a week, for 30 to 45 minutes each time.

You can also turn walking into a HIIT workout by alternating periods of jogging with periods of slower walking.

Strength Training

This is a type of weight-bearing activity using weights, resistance bands, or your own body weight, in which your muscles are challenged to work harder each time they're exercised. It develops not only muscle but also bone strength, therefore preventing osteoporosis as you get older.

A 2009 study published in the *European Journal of Applied Physiology* involving forty-two perimenopausal women offered proof of the benefits of strength training. The women worked out with weights for 60 minutes three times a week. Each week they got stronger, developed more muscle, and strengthened their VO2max, a measurement of the body's ability to consume oxygen. The better your VO2max, the more oxygen goes to your muscles for a more intense exercise effort.

Findings from the Study of Women's Health Across the Nation (SWAN), a study of ten thousand women as they go through menopause, showed that 20 to 30 percent of forty- to fifty-five-year-olds had difficulty performing simple physical tasks such as climbing a flight of stairs or carrying grocery bags around the block. Even putting clothes on over your head or clasping your bra strap can become difficult. If women are that weak then, what will happen to them at eighty?

Fortunately, various studies show that engaging in just two strength-training workouts a week increases strength in women over fifty quite significantly. The sooner you start, the better you'll feel and look!

Lift weights, use strength-training machines, use bands, or perform body weight exercises at least two days a week. Do one set each of ten to twelve moves that strengthen your major muscle groups — arms, shoulders, chest, back, abdominals, hips, and legs. If you're beginning, choose a lighter weight you can lift at least 15 to 20 times. Once this gets comfortable and you are over the soreness, increase the weights to where you can do a maximum of only 10 to 12 reps.

Yoga

The word "yoga" actually refers to a union of body, mind, and spirit, an alignment of the physical and nonphysical parts of yourself. It's not an overstatement: If you practice yoga, not only will you find that your health and well-being improve, but every area of your life will benefit.

Yoga is particularly important for stopping or reversing osteoporosis, which can strike during the years after menopause. A 2016 study, published in *Topics in Geriatric Rehabilitation,* found that 80 percent of older participants, most of whom had osteoporosis or its precursor, osteopenia (low bone density), who practiced certain yoga poses for just 12 minutes a day, holding each pose for 30 seconds, improved the bone density in their spine and femurs.

I wasn't too surprised by these findings. Yoga plays a vital role in preventing fractures by building stability, flexibility, and agility. This means you're less likely to fall and break something — and if you do start to fall, your flexibility is likely to help you catch yourself.

Yoga is a wonderful stress reliever and health builder — a fact proven by hundreds of studies. A 2017 review of forty-two studies, published in *Psychoneuroendocrinology*, offered some dramatic proof of yoga's power. Yoga was shown to do all of the following:

- Reduced levels of evening cortisol. This was significant, since we want cortisol to be low in the evening so we can get a good night's sleep and let the body repair itself. Many people who are stressed out are victims of high cortisol at night.

- Lowered blood pressure, resting heart rate, and LDL cholesterol—signs of a healthy cardiovascular system.

- Elevated heart rate variability (HRV)—the beat-to-beat fluctuations in heart rate. When you're feeling calm and relaxed, HRV goes up, and you can more effortlessly manage stress. In healthy people, HRV is high. A high HRV is a positive factor in cardiovascular health, your fitness level, even your longevity. I have found consistently low HRV in clients under chronic stress and with PTSD.

- Reduced fasting blood glucose—which means blood sugar and insulin are under good control.

Yoga is absolutely for everyone! Classes are available at practically all gyms, fitness centers, and community centers, so you should be able to easily enroll in a class that meets your needs and level of experience. No matter how time-crunched you are, you can create time for yoga. In fact, yoga will create more time for you.

Aquatic Resistance Training

This activity involves the use of resistance devices or elastic bands designed for use in a pool, usually performed under the guidance of an instructor. It can be very easy on the joints, and is an excellent form of exercise if you have osteoarthritis or other joint issues, or want to build strength.

A study in the *European Journal of Physiology* reported that when forty-six postmenopausal women took part in a twenty-four-week aquatic resistance class, they lost body fat, increased muscle, and lowered their blood pressure.

Water exercise is a great way to get fit, especially if you don't like to swim. Check to see if your gym, health spa, or local YMCA offers aquatic exercise classes.

Dance

You're never too old to kick up your heels—and get fit in the process, plus improve your quality of life. According to a 2016 study published in *Menopause,* fifty-two sedentary postmenopausal women were randomly assigned to receive either dance therapy or participate in a non-dance control group. The dancers completed two months of dance therapy, three sessions weekly. By the end of the study, the women in the dance group had improved their balance, mobility, cardiac fitness, flexibility, and energy levels significantly, compared to the control group (which had no such improvements).

Dancing is also good for mental health, because the act of remembering steps and coordinating them to the music is an excellent way to "exercise" your brain.

Many YMCAs, community centers, and gyms offer dance and dance exercise classes. Consider joining up and being a part of the fun.

So there you have it—lots of ways to not only get more fit but also help rebalance your hormones for weight control. Fitting some daily movement into your life is one of the best ways to support both physical health and mental health. With the combo of both, achieving better hormone balance may be more possible than you think.

Whatever type of exercise appeals to you, please, please get active! Numerous studies demonstrate that many of the changes—both physical and mental—that we associate with aging and menopause are partly the result of inactivity. Many of the women I have worked with over the years—women who began exercising before and during menopause—tell me that it changed their lives. Let exercise change yours!

Chapter 10

The Clean 16

. . . .

There is one more component of my Keto-Green 16 plan that is, like exercise, not diet related. It includes daily rituals for positive reinforcement—actions I call my Clean 16. They will help you stay the course and value yourself like never before. Use them in conjunction with my plan.

Practice Daily Affirmations

Each day, begin with affirmations to set a course for success. Tell yourself something positive. Repeat it a few times, write it down, text it to yourself, or take a screenshot, and look at it throughout the day. With enough repetition, they will become reality for you. Make them in the present tense such as "I am" or "I have," not "I will" or "I could." Here are my favorite affirmations:

I am happy and joyful.
I am content.
I am energetic.

I am productive.
I am social and friendly.
I am alert.
My mind is focused.
I feel good about my body.
I believe in myself; I can be everything I want to be.
I am strong, full of energy and confidence.
I deserve to look and feel great.
If it challenges me, it changes me.

I always focus on positive "I can do this" affirmations. I don't want my happiness to be contingent on numbers on a scale; rather, I want it to be based on what I accomplish toward making myself a better person, creating better relationships, and making the world a better place today. I remember that I'm the only one who can upset myself, and no one else has that power over me.

Saying affirmations each day helps you embrace them. Your mind and body start believing in you. You will make better decisions. You'll see a difference and become more happy, joyful, content, social, productive, friendly, and focused. Try it for a few weeks, and you'll see what I mean.

Keep a Journal

Many of us in the medical field focus on compassion and care. This can be both rewarding and depleting. To offset the depletion part, I began expressing my thoughts and emotions in a journal.

Journaling turned out to be a valuable resource to help me tend to my own well-being and support my health. Research has found that journaling reduces blood pressure, improves mood, and boosts focus and productivity. It has become a daily practice for me—sometimes super-easy, other times not so much. I love to journal in the morning while sipping my Keto Coffee or Keto Tea; I express what I'm grateful for and set my intentions for the day.

The gratitude component is key. It makes you not only a happier person but a healthier one as well. The expression of gratitude improves mental health, reduces anxiety, and helps you sleep better. Giving gratitude is a great way to create more oxytocin and just feel better overall. Grateful people tend to be happier, more positive, and more satisfied with their lives, compared to people who walk through life without an attitude of gratitude.

Take five to fifteen minutes and do some gratitude journaling every day. Ask yourself these questions: "What am I grateful for? What have I done to nourish my body and mind today? Where did I see love today?"

Just sit quietly and allow yourself to feel the sentiment of gratefulness for all the blessings in life. Journaling replenishes your mind and body with the strength to take care of yourself and others for whom you have responsibility.

Practice Meditation

We know from scientific studies and research that meditation is beneficial to your body, mind, and spirit. I learned this from a trip I took several years ago, when I got to stay at a monastery tucked away in the woods. I was completely disconnected from the media, world events, and office happenings. It was tremendously healing and upgrading to my quality of life.

But you don't have to travel to a monastery to meditate. You can do it in the privacy of our own home or the sanctuary of your backyard. Simply do a bit of meditative reflection by asking yourself, "How can I be more loving, receive more love, or laugh more?"

Meditation helps you achieve your fitness goals too. When you meditate, imagine yourself as you want to look a few months from now. See yourself in a swimsuit, outfit, or dress that used to fit you. Bring these images to your mind exactly as you want them to unfold. Include as many details as you can. Focus on your vision and how it makes you feel, and push away any doubts by making positive statements to yourself. Your inner vision and feelings will give shape to your desires and make them real. I call this "feelingiza-tion."

Compartmentalize

Do you feel like your life is spinning out of control? Are you jug-gling so many demands that you can't keep up? Do you sometimes feel like you're a pinball machine on tilt?

I've noticed some of these signs at times, and when I do, I stop and pay attention. I know I'm headed for a crash-and-burn when I get overscheduled with too many speaking engagements and proj-ects. There's a lot of inner chaos I then have to deal with.

A practice I learned some time ago was to compartmentalize. When worries creep in, direct them to a designated time when you'll give consideration to those thoughts and honor them. For example, when I have a problem that I'm worried about and thoughts come up to distract me during my day, I simply say, "Not now. Move to 8:15 or 8:30 P.M. I will get to you later." This allows me to focus and have better productivity throughout the day.

Many of us may have experienced trauma, or maybe we're cur-rently in a repeating behavior pattern and just need help to break that cycle. Compartmentalizing helps.

Take in Nature

Walk out the door each day, spend time in nature, and give yourself a moment to pause and notice the beauty of our world. At your coffee break, take a few minutes to gaze out a window at your beau-tiful surroundings. Take deep belly breaths while doing this. This practice will help you calm your sympathetic nervous system (which can make you feel stressed when out of balance), increase the activity of your parasympathetic nervous system, helping you chill, and increase heart rate variability. It's a perfect reset practice.

People who take nature walks with others are less likely to report feeling depressed and stressed and more likely to score higher on assessments of mental and emotional well-being than their non-nature-walking peers, according to a large British study published in 2019 in the *International Journal of Environmental Research and Public Health*. The findings added to a growing body of research that suggests exposure to nature, especially when combined with walking, improves psychological well-being.

Before sixty-two-year-old Shaynel started living the Keto-Green lifestyle, she was carrying around ten pounds of stubborn body fat and had brain fog and depression. She believed that her depression was linked to seasonal affective disorder (SAD), a mood disorder that's related to changes in seasons and limited sunlight. SAD begins and ends at about the same times every year and is correlated with drearier, darker days during the year.

Shaynel recounted to me one depressing winter day when she was headed home at about 3:30 P.M. Dark and gloomy, the afternoon was freezing cold. Even so, she parked her car at a lake and just walked around for ten minutes, taking in the views and fresh air. She recalled how recharged and energized that had made her feel. Her mood immediately lifted.

The experience was so life-changing that Shaynel made a habit of getting outside and connecting with nature on a daily basis, even if only for a few minutes. She found that her entire view of winter changed—rather than seeing it as only dreary and dreadful, she came to relish its beauty and enjoyed how being outside and capturing the changing light made her feel, almost as if she were somehow resetting some internal rhythm in her body. No matter what, even if the day is freezing cold, Shaynel now ensures she gets some time out-of-doors each day. Her depression and brain fog have vanished.

She knows that this practice, now a permanent habit, also helps her get a great night's sleep. As for her weight, Shaynel lost those ten pounds very quickly. After doing Keto-Green, she needed to buy a new bra and dress. She was a bit shocked that her usual size 36 or 38 bra was now a 34, and she was fitting into smaller-size dresses.

Like Shaynel, I always feel better after a walk on the beach or a hike in the woods, admiring the trees, the flowers, the sky, or the ocean, and it has a calming, alkalinizing effect on my body. Yes, I walk partly to stay in shape, but when I'm walking in God's creation, it is more about grounding.

Pamper Yourself with Essential Oils

Maybe you've already discovered the power of essential oils. That's great, because various studies show that they can soothe us and ease the psychological symptoms of menopause, such as anxiety, depression, and mood swings. They also help young and middle-aged women relax. Some act as phytoestrogens because they have components related to the sex hormone estrogen.

We're all concerned about tummy fat. Essential oils may be helpful here too. In 2007 Korean researchers divided women into two groups. One group received one hour of whole-body massage every week for six weeks. They also massaged their own abdomen twice a day, five days a week, for six weeks. They used different kinds of oil. The experimental group applied 3 percent grapefruit oil, cypress, and three other kinds of essential oils. The control group used grapeseed oil. Their waist circumference was measured before and after the experiment.

In the experimental group, belly fat just under the skin as well as waist circumference significantly decreased, compared to the control group. Body image—how much they liked their appearance—was significantly better in the experimental group after aromatherapy massage than in the control group.

The researchers said: "These results suggest that aromatherapy massage could be utilized as an effective intervention to reduce abdominal subcutaneous fat, waist circumference, and to improve body image in post-menopausal women." Interesting, isn't it? There's a lot we can do to get a flat belly!

The following chart lists the benefits of commonly used essential oils.

ESSENTIAL OIL	BENEFITS
Basil oil	Contains compounds similar to estrogen and helps balance this hormone
Clary sage oil	Eases hot flashes, helps thyroid function, reduces depression, and lowers stress levels
Evening primrose oil	Relieves breast tenderness when taken orally
Geranium oil	Balances hormones, improves dry skin, and boosts mood
Lavender oil	Enhances relaxation and sleep quality; balances hormones
Neroli oil	Enhances estrogen balance and reduces blood pressure when inhaled; acts as an anti-inflammatory agent
Peppermint oil	Relieves hot flashes and menstrual pain
Rose oil	Improves uterine function
Vitex agnus-castus oil	Helps improve many symptoms of PMS, perimenopause, and menopause; helps infertility in women; reduces chance of miscarriage in women who are low in progesterone

If you're considering combining a number of these oils to help you deal with various symptoms, here are some ways to get the most benefits:

- Make your own body moisturizer by combining 5 to 8 drops of your preferred essential oil with a carrier oil such as sweet almond oil. Rub into your skin two to three times daily. You can also use a liquid carrier oil to make your own massage or bath oil.

- Place 2 drops of your preferred oil on tissue paper and hold it under your nose. Inhale its fragrance when you are experiencing menopausal symptoms.

- Combine 2 to 10 drops of oil with 2 ounces of purified water. Place the mixture in a spray bottle and then spray it in your home.

- Combine 8 drops oil with ½ cup coconut milk and pour the mixture into a hot bath.

Cherish Family Relationships

Nothing is more magical to me than spending time with my four beautiful daughters. Although I have lots of things going on, I make sure they come first.

Try to carve out time each day to connect with those around you. Making time for your loved ones increases oxytocin in your body, with all the positive health benefits that brings, and reduces stress. An easy suggestion? Don't watch TV during dinner; instead, sit down with your partner or family and share in everyone's day. Make every day a truly special one for all of the relationships in your life. Ask each other about what you are excited about and what you are concerned about. Try asking where they saw or felt love today too.

Having said that, I don't want to leave you with the impression that my family life is drama free; after all, I have four daughters. I can remember asking two of them, "When will you stop hating me?" They responded, "We don't hate you, Mom!" Oh, but it sure felt like it at times!

Now, that may be a function of mom-daughter dynamics during the teenage years, but it was also during my menopause transition, when I was in my mid- to late forties—before I figured out my Keto-Green way of living. Once I focused on self-care, all my relationships improved. I say this to encourage you to put yourself first with loving self-care. When you take care of yourself, those around you, the ones you've been putting first and have been sacrificing yourself for, will benefit greatly. Now my daughters and I have the best relationships of our lives, and I know I am setting a better example for them now than I was as their haggard mom back then.

Reframe Your Goals

After repeatedly setting many New Year's resolutions and typically breaking them after a few months (or days), I decided a few years ago to ditch them in place of what I call Love Your Life Goals. Setting these goals involves four simple steps:

Step 1: Kindly accept where you are right now.
Step 2: Reflect on what you loved about yesterday, last week, and last year.
Step 3: Clarify what you love about your life right now and what you want to find more of (the answers will be your Love Your Life Goals).
Step 4: Write down your Love Your Life Goals.

Your goals will be unique to you; one of my goals was to have even better relationships with my daughters and more quality family time together.

After working out what I want my goals to be, I set them into a workable timeline of daily, weekly, and longer-term deadlines. This helps me stay focused and chart my progress.

Put Yourself First

As a doctor and a mom, I was always taking care of everyone else. My own needs used to take a backseat. I needed a course correction in order to feel whole again.

I started by modifying my diet. I pursued a better diet, and ended up creating my Keto-Green plan. It was like magic! I had boundless energy. I dropped pounds quickly. My menopause symptoms vanished. My brain fog lifted, so I was able to make better decisions. My stress levels got better. I knew I was on to something *big*, something that turned my life around.

I encourage you to prioritize your own self-care, stay Keto-Green, and live the Keto-Green lifestyle. You'll stay slim, sane, and sexy, feel more energetic, revive your libido, look and feel younger—and transform your life in ways you can't even yet imagine. Take care of yourself now, and you will cement habits that will serve you well into your golden years.

Putting yourself first also means being good and kind to yourself and not beating yourself up when you suffer, fail, or feel inadequate. In short, it means treating yourself the way you would your best friend. Self-compassion is healing at many levels. It can bring you out of a depression and change your entire body chemistry by flooding your system with feel-good hormones.

A simple exercise is to look at yourself in the mirror, into your eyes, and speak loving truths to your precious self and do some positive coaching. Try saying: "You are so beautiful and just wonderfully created. You have the potential to do anything you really want to do. You are healthy, loving, kind, and good," and continue from there. You may feel self-conscious, but you'll also find that speaking kindly and encouragingly to yourself feels good. This is a powerful practice.

Self-monitor

Research shows that if we make ourselves accountable by self-monitoring, we'll be more successful at losing weight. Self-monitoring is the ability to both observe and evaluate your behavior and progress. There are lots of ways to self-monitor:

Test your pH and ketones regularly.
Monitor your blood sugar with Libre Freestyle or finger sticks periodically.
Measure your waist.
Hop on the scale.
Monitor your blood panels periodically, especially hsCRP, HbA1c, DHEA-S, and vitamin D.

Remember that journal you're keeping? It's a great place to record your self-monitoring results. That way you can track your progress and stay mindful of how your actions positively or negatively impact your ability to succeed. It can even serve as a warning device if your numbers are sliding off track.

With your milestones written down in black and white, you can periodically evaluate your progress, flipping back to previous weeks and gauging how well you're sticking to your plan. If you're slacking off and picking up old bad habits, make course corrections to get back on track.

Take the One Next Right Step

Often the journey toward self-improvement can feel overwhelming. Here's my solution. Ask yourself: "What's the one next right step I can take today?" It might be as simple as eating a Keto-Green lunch, putting more green veggies on your plate, going to the gym tonight, fitting in an intermittent fast, pampering yourself with a massage or facial, or writing in your journal.

Just take the one next right step. This has kept me from trying to outrun my past and obsessing over the traumas, griefs, pain, failed relationships, and rejections I—like everyone else—have had. Looking back has a way of pulling us back. As I like to say, God gave us eyes in front of our face to look forward, not back.

Tap into the Healing Power of Community

When I'm frazzled by stress and the busyness of life, I turn to family and friends. I gather my loved ones, call my relatives who live out of town, or just get together with my friends. With each hug, ripple of laugher, and gesture of encouragement, my stress eases and I feel better.

As it turns out, these feelings—and these relationships—have long-term benefits. According to mounting evidence, positive connections create better health, with dividends that include a healthier heart and a longer life.

One reason is that being connected produces oxytocin. We make more of it when we feel love; when we share warm emotional contact of any type; when we give birth and cradle our newborn; and when we have sex. It's an anti-aging hormone too, vital to healing and restoring hormonal balance.

The less oxytocin we make, the more free radicals we generate and the more susceptible we are to illness. But the opposite is true too: Being connected helps boost the immune system and prevent disease. Oxytocin also causes the cells lining artery walls to relax. When this happens, blood pressure normalizes—which ultimately means protection against heart attack and stroke. To stimulate all of these wonderful things, we must be connected to a loving community. Community is where we heal.

Here are some ideas to help you strengthen your connections and make the most of community in your life:

- Say yes to invitations and opportunities as they present themselves. We can say yes too often and overcommit, so be cautious. But do make an effort to socialize. Because of stress and hormone changes, many of us can lean toward isolation. But a healthy and balanced social life is beneficial.

- Don't wait for invitations either. Take the initiative and invite a new or old friend over for a cup of coffee, or meet up somewhere for a drink or walk.

- Nurture friendships. Oxytocin promotes a friend-seeking response in women. Women need other women—we guide each other, console each other, and celebrate with each other. The long-running Harvard-based Nurses' Health Study found that the more close friends a woman has, the less likely she is to suffer physical ills as she ages. In fact, not having at least one true confidant can ultimately be as detrimental to your health as being a heavy smoker!

- Join a support group. I'd suggest my Keto-Green Facebook community. It is an amazing group of women who share their trials and triumphs, ask questions about hormones and

health, and offer support and encouragement to other
women practicing my Keto-Green lifestyle.

- Be generous. Giving is a way to increase oxytocin. Just try it
and see. I regularly volunteer at church with the kids'
groups. I also created a foundation in honor of my late son,
called the Garrett V. Bivens Foundation. Through it, we've
done some very beautiful things, including teaching tots to
swim and helping to found the House of Hope, a safe home
and rehabilitation center for girls who've been caught up in
human trafficking.

So tap into community. All the longest-living people in the world
have this in common: a good social life and community. Both will
give you a big dose of happiness and health. It's a prescription that
works.

Take Stock

I'm in my early fifties, and I think a lot about how I want to feel in
my seventies and beyond. Years ago, being in your seventies meant
being old. Not anymore! With our ability to reverse the aging process, ninety is the new seventy. We are living longer, and by taking
action with diet, supplements, exercise, and mind-body work, we
can slow down aging and join in the remarkable revolution in
healthcare that emphasizes prevention over treatment. If you're a
woman in your forties, fifties, sixties, or older, ask yourself: "What
do I need to do *now* to add quality, productive years to my life?"

Write Thank-You Notes

I'm not talking emails or texts! I'm talking about taking pen to actual paper and writing notes to people to let them know I appreciate
them, whether that is because of something they did or simply be-

cause of who they are to me. I will do this in my morning meditation time, sometimes challenging myself to do this ten days in a
row.

There is something very gratifying about sitting down with paper
and pen in hand and actually writing a well-thought-out thank-you
note from the heart. It has a healing effect on my body, mind, and
spirit.

View Yourself Positively

How do you feel about yourself today? I have found a large per-
centage of people see themselves in a negative fashion, in some way.
Maybe they think they are too fat or too thin. Maybe they don't
see themselves as "enough" of something—social enough, pretty
enough, vibrant enough, or sexy enough. They may have a health
issue or symptoms that they've just accepted as "the way things
are" instead of trying to get healthier through lifestyle changes.

I believe that when we get in touch with how we really feel about
ourselves and the world around us, it helps us to confront our issues and deal with them better. So if you are feeling fat, maybe it's
because you're eating a lot of sugar, carbs, grains, or white stuff.

If you keep allowing negative beliefs to drive your behavior,
you'll throw roadblocks in the way of your success every time. The
way you remove these roadblocks is to first recognize the effects of
these beliefs in your life and then rewrite the underlying script.
Work on releasing negative beliefs about yourself so that you can
step into brilliance. You're worthy of all the blessings coming your
way.

Celebrate Immediately

Celebrate little wins along the way—losing a few pounds, going to
the gym twice this week, getting rid of junk food in your kitchen,
drinking lots of pure water, and so forth.

In building new habits, it helps to reward yourself in positive ways—even tiny ones, like giving yourself a thumbs-up, smiling in the mirror, getting some new lipstick, or just telling yourself you did a great job.

Achieving both short- and long-term goals requires ongoing motivation, which can be supported by regular infusions of feel-good dopamine, the ultimate pleasure and motivation "drug." Good news: You don't have to buy it or inject it. Dopamine is in your body naturally. You just have to supercharge it. Rewarding yourself and celebrating your accomplishments as soon as they happen causes surges of dopamine in your body.

Creating a healthy lifestyle can be challenging. Expect that at some point you'll struggle with motivation. That's normal. Use my Clean 16 to inspire you and keep you on track through this plan. With these strategies in mind, and with commitment, determination, and belief in yourself, there's no reason you can't achieve astounding success in sixteen days.

Chapter 11

Day 17 and Beyond

. . . .

Looking at the slim, sculpted frame of Inez, a participant in my online program Magic Menopause, it's difficult to believe that this lovely lady lost more than 100 pounds—and kept it off—by going Keto-Green at age fifty-seven.

She once had to hide her body in baggy clothes. She had no energy. Her hair was falling out in clumps. Her hormones were completely out of balance. Her menopause symptoms were unbearable. But Inez signed up for my program and overhauled her diet and lifestyle. She stuck with it for months and months. Now she's back in dresses she hasn't worn in thirty years. She looks younger at fifty-seven than she did at twenty-seven (a lot of it has to do with her hair coming back). And she feels like she's gotten her life back.

Inez achieved huge, important accomplishments, something a lot of people fail to do because they don't have the right program or direction. But now you have the right program that will keep you healthy and in shape.

Inez is my poster lady for how to do Keto-Green for life. Which is what you must do in order to reach and maintain your happy weight. You can't return to your former bad eating habits, because those habits disrupted your hormones, which helped bring about the weight gain and the unhealthy lifestyle in the first place.

If you still have more weight to lose, it is perfectly fine—and indeed a good idea—to spend another sixteen days on this plan, using it in cycles until you reach your goal. Or you can switch to a more liberal version of the plan, a maintenance version (outlined in this chapter), and return to the sixteen-day program every now and then to get you to your weight goal. In other words, you can cycle on and off Keto-Green 16 as needed.

The guidelines that follow will help you keep the weight off while letting you enjoy yourself a little more, expand your food choices, and even eat freely with your favorite foods by feasting on certain days.

Go Beyond the 16 Foods: Expand Your Diet to Include More Keto-Green Foods

After the sixteen-day plan, feel free to expand your food choices while still staying Keto-Green. Here's a list of foods, categorized by alkalinity and carb content, to focus on.

Vegetables

Highly Alkaline/Low-Carb Vegetables
Beet greens
Cucumber
Kelp and other sea vegetables
Keto Alkaline Broth (page 221)
Maca
Parsley
Radishes (black)
Spinach
Sprouts, all types

Highly Alkaline/Moderate-Carb Vegetables
Dandelion greens
Jicama
Kale
Turnip greens

Moderately Alkaline/Low-Carb Vegetables
Arugula
Asparagus
Bamboo shoots
Basil
Broccoli
Cauliflower
Celery
Chives
Collard greens
Endive
Green cabbage
Lettuce
Mustard greens
Peppers (hot)
Pumpkin
Radishes (red, white)
Savoy cabbage
Spring greens
Tomato
Turnips
Watercress
White cabbage

Moderately Alkaline/Moderate-Carb Vegetables
Artichoke
Garlic
Green beans

Okra
Soybeans
Squash (winter)

Mildly Alkaline/Low-Carb Vegetables
Bell peppers
Bok choy
Brussels sprouts
Eggplant
Herbs and spices
Kohlrabi
Mushrooms
Pickles (not sweetened)
Squash (summer)
Zucchini

Mildly Alkaline/Moderate-Carb Vegetables
Beets
Carrots
Leeks
Onions (red, white)
Peas
Red cabbage
Rhubarb
Rutabaga

Fruits

Highly Alkaline/Moderate-Carb Fruits
Cantaloupe
Melons, other
Watermelon

Digestive Support Fruits
Mango
Papaya
Pineapple

Moderately Alkaline/Low-Carb Fruits
Berries
Carob

Moderately Alkaline/Moderate-Carb Fruits
Apricot
Avocado
Lemon
Lime

Mildly Alkaline/Low-Carb Fruits
Coconut, fresh
Olives

Mildly Alkaline/Moderate-Carb Fruits
Grapefruit

Moderately Alkaline/Low-Carb Nuts and Seeds
Chia seeds
Hemp hearts

Mildly Alkaline/Low-Carb Nuts and Seeds
Almond butter
Almond milk
Almonds
Brazil nuts
Pine nuts
Sesame seeds

Fats and Oils

Moderately Alkaline Fats and Oils
Flaxseed oil

Mildly Alkaline Fats and Oils
Avocado oil
Coconut oil

Fish oil
MCT oil
Olive oil, extra-virgin
Sesame oil

Mildly Acid/Low-Carb Nuts and Seeds
Cashews
Coconut, dried
Macadamias
Pecans
Pistachios
Pumpkin seeds
Sunflower seeds
Walnuts

Proteins

Highly Acid/Low-Carb Protein
Beef
Bison (buffalo)
Chicken
Eggs, organic and cage-free
Lamb
Pork
Rabbit
Turkey
Venison

Alkaline Vegan Proteins
Beans, all varieties
Lentils
Tempeh
Tofu

Moderately Acid/Low-Carb Protein
Fish
Shellfish

Plan Your Keto-Green Meals

My maintenance Keto-Green diet adheres to the following ratios: 55–70 percent fats, 5–15 percent carbohydrates, and 15–25 percent protein. On a plate, this means greens and alkalinizing vegetables account for 75 percent of the surface area. Proteins make up a palm-size amount, approximately 4 to 6 ounces. Then imagine a circle in the center of the plate, which equals approximately ¼ cup healthy fats, such as avocados, nuts, or olive oil. For breakfast, feel free to have a Keto-Green shake every morning, one of the smoothies in the recipe section, or any of my Keto-Green breakfast recipes. Try to eat this way most days of the week.

Enjoy Breakfast, Lunch, and Dinner

Although many of my clients typically eat two meals per day, continuing with thirteen-to-sixteen-hour intermittent fasts, you can eat three meals a day, if desired. Always include some kind of protein at every meal—vegetarian proteins, eggs, fish, shellfish, poultry, or grass-fed meat—along with your alkalinizing vegetables. Also, eat moderate amounts of protein.

Remember: if you can pick it, peel it, fish it, hunt it, milk it, or grow it, you can eat it on my plan for the most part.

Consider portion control. Try to switch up meal portions so you eat lighter in the evening. Eat breakfast like a king, lunch like a prince, and dinner like a pauper—or a college kid with a maxed-out credit card. Make breakfast your largest meal of the day, but not the typical high-glycemic, unhealthy-fat-heavy American breakfast consisting of a stack of pancakes, two eggs, some bacon or a sausage biscuit, and a glass of orange juice. Make your choices from low-glycemic options, or skip all the cooking and do a protein smoothie mixed with a few berries, almond milk, Dr. Anna Cabeca Keto-Green meal replacement, and so forth. Consider adding kale, spinach, or other greens to a blended smoothie for an extra nutritional punch; you'll be amazed to find that when they're blended with other ingredients you won't taste the greens.

I think that you should eat your fruit instead of drinking it. And when you do have fruit, choose lower-glycemic options such as seasonal berries and melons, or continue enjoying the digestive support fruits mango, papaya, and pineapple with your evening meals.

A lower-glycemic breakfast means less spiking of your blood sugar, improved metabolism, and less hunger before lunch and throughout the day.

Lunch should be of average size—not the size of either breakfast or dinner, but in between. Have some protein, a veggie or two, maybe even some brown rice on occasion.

Now for dinner! Choose something light, nothing big—go for high-quality protein and healthy fats, and avoid the sugars and carbs. Ideally, finish eating before 7 P.M. Realize that sugar, carbs, and unhealthy fats make you sick and fat. Healthy fats, proteins, and produce make you healthy!

The caveat to my three-meals-a-day rule is when you're doing intermittent prolonged fasts. As you become more practiced at being Keto-Green, you may comfortably be able to have just one to two meals a day. Personally, I occasionally like to combine my Keto-Green shake with my lunch meal but then have nothing else until dinner. Take your time and don't push it, because if you get too aggressive too fast with intermittent fasting, the hunger hormone ghrelin can surge and sabotage your good intentions. Also, I will often flip my meals and have a healthy Keto-Green lunch and then a Keto-Green shake for dinner. This is really helpful as a reset when the number on the scale is creeping up, when I am feeling bloated, when I've just gotten back from vacation, or after a weekend of extra indulgences.

Eat Keto-Green Clean

Stop eating from boxes, bags, and cans. Stay away from the processed foods; try to eat raw and minimally processed as much as possible. Eat clean meats, meaning grass-fed or free-range, raised without antibiotics, steroids, or hormones. Consume pesticide-free, organic vegetables and fruits. Avoid fast foods and cook at home when you can.

If you eat fruit, go for the lower-carb varieties, and keep the number of servings at two or fewer a day.

As for grains, limit these to two servings a day max. Choose low-glycemic options such as brown rice and quinoa.

Watch out for gluten. It is an inflammatory protein found in foods made from wheat and related grain species, including barley and rye. (Occasionally oats can be contaminated with gluten as well, though they are naturally gluten free.) You should eliminate or reduce your gluten intake to assist in metabolism, improve your digestive health, and reduce inflammation.

Be sure to include healthy fats like olive oil, avocados, nuts, seeds, and coconut oil. They help with hormone balance, keep you feeling satiated, and support hormone production. Fats to include are avocados, egg yolks, homemade mayo, homemade salad dressings, Hollandaise sauce, nuts, olives, grass-fed butter or ghee, and coconut and olive oils.

When shopping for the foods you plan to eat, make the majority of your choices selections that you'll find on the periphery of your supermarket. There you will find produce and proteins. Be aware that 80–90 percent of the foods located along the inner aisles are packaged and processed.

In short, always build your meals around Keto-Green whole foods. This is one of the smartest moves you can make to keep your weight under control. Some occasional rice and quinoa may be fine for you, but be aware that if you are struggling at all, completely eliminate them.

Stay Hydrated to Stay Slim

We hear a lot of advice about the importance of drinking water, but did you know that adequate hydration also helps you keep the weight off?

It's true: hydration is a weight maintenance strategy—for a number of reasons.

- According to a study published in the *Journal of Human Nutrition and Dietetics,* drinking more water causes you to eat fewer calories and less sugar, salt, and cholesterol. For the study, researchers from the University of Illinois at Urbana-Champaign interviewed 18,311 adults about everything they ate and drank on two different occasions, between three and ten days apart. After analyzing answers, the researchers observed that an increase in daily plain water consumption by between 1 and 3 cups was associated with a reduction in daily total energy intake by between 69 and 206 calories. That might sound insignificant, but 206 extra calories a day adds up to a pound of fat gained in about seventeen days.

- Water is an appetite suppressant. To help you keep pounds from piling back on, drink 16 ounces of water thirty minutes prior to a meal, and you won't overeat at meals. You may even lose a little weight. That's what happened to a group of adults age fifty-five and older when they drank 2 cups of water before meals. They automatically lost nearly five pounds in twelve weeks without even changing their diets. This study was reported in *Obesity* in 2007. So if you drink some water half an hour before your meals, your body will have a sensation of being full, and you will automatically eat less.

- Adequate hydration boosts metabolism. Because your body is largely powered by water, drinking enough water actually raises your metabolism and the rate at which you burn fat. Cold water is especially good at this, because your body must spend more energy to bring your body temperature back to normal equilibrium. Keeping your metabolism high is key to keeping your body at its happy weight.

- Water detoxifies your body. Water and kidneys work together to get rid of toxins and electrolytes that are prejudicial to the body. It starts with the kidneys filtering our blood to eliminate the toxins. Good blood flow is what makes this happen, and blood flow is optimal when the proper amount of water is running through the system. If there isn't enough water available, the toxins will not be expelled. This can generate different types of disorders and even diseases.

- Water increases muscle performance. When you sweat through exercise, more fluid is needed to keep your body functioning at its best. Staying hydrated during physical activity will help you perform at your optimal level—which in turn translates into staying in great shape and keeping pounds from coming back.

- Water elevates your mood. Brain function is directly affected by hydration. Your mood, memory, and ability to process information can all be elevated by drinking enough healthy fluids.

- Water boosts energy. If you're feeling lethargic, this may be a sign of dehydration. Consuming water throughout the day can boost your energy levels, which in turn can motivate you to stay active and accomplish your goals.

Keep an Eye on Ketosis

Achieving ketosis is still important after you reach your happy weight. Try to stay in ketosis most days of the week, especially Monday through Thursday or Friday. Restrict your carbohydrate intake (basically, no bread, cereals, pasta, grains, or other starchy or sugary carbs). A good guideline is to keep your carbs at around 40 grams a day or less.

Make Intermittent Fasting a Part of Your Lifestyle

Now that you've set your course on a healthy regimen, continue to integrate fasting into your life. Fasting is like painting your house, an additional protective layer on your investment. You don't want to paint the house if you haven't yet dealt with the wood rot, right? You need a good foundation, which the Keto-Green 16 plan provides. Fasting helps solidify your efforts, protecting your investment in your health and your happy weight.

Sometimes people think that intermittent fasting is a fancy way of saying starving yourself to lose weight. This couldn't be further from the truth. Intermittent fasting is a pattern of eating that can be sustained for a lifetime.

Over the years, I've continued to practice intermittent fasting. One of the main reasons it helps me keep my weight off is because it helps to reduce the amount of time I spend preparing food—and ultimately the amount of food I eat. The less food we eat, the more weight we lose.

Thus I regularly do intermittent fasting throughout the week to control my weight, with fasts of sixteen hours between dinner and breakfast—sometimes longer, sometimes shorter. Then I eat two good Keto-Green meals and possibly one light meal or protein shake in an eight-hour window, without snacking. Then about once a month I also do a water fast that lasts twenty-four to seventy-two hours (see page 78). I encourage you to do both strategies as well, and I know you'll love the weight-control benefits.

Let me just emphasize that we want *healthy* fasting. Some women take it too far, which leads to them feeling unwell. When you are fasting, you need to be doubly sure that you are taking in the nutrients that your body needs, nourishing your body at the cellular level. (Remember, if you are under a doctor's care for diabetes, if you are pregnant or nursing, or if you have other health issues, you shouldn't undertake an extended fast without first getting clearance from your doctor.)

Enjoy Occasional Feasts

Occasional feasting with your favorite foods exemplifies a sensible and moderate way of eating. You can stick to a fairly strict Keto-Green diet during the week but give yourself some leeway occasionally on a weekend or for a special social event. Having treats can actually encourage you and keep you loving this lifestyle. Then come Monday it's back to vegetables, good fats, and protein. You're compensating by going Keto-Green during the week. If you keep up your exercise program, there's no way you're going to regain pounds when you feast like this. You may even lose weight!

That said, if you see the scale register five pounds over your happy weight, go right back on the sixteen-day plan. It will get you back to that weight faster and is a fantastic weight-control tool you now have in your Keto-Green bag of tricks.

Also, use your feast day to discover more about your reaction to food. If you do experience food sensitivity symptoms after eating a particular food, such as swelling, congestion, headache, bloating, weight gain, or general malaise, then stay away from that food. Also, if you are suffering from medical conditions you are trying to reverse, then stay 100 percent compliant with Keto-Green and stick to a Keto-Green feast day periodically.

Live the Keto-Green Lifestyle

The reality about Keto-Green eating is that it involves more than following a food plan. It's about making a commitment to living a Keto-Green lifestyle—a new way of living.

There are several Keto-Green lifestyle principles that I'll summarize here. Their common denominator is that they help maintain your body in an alkaline state (the healthiest physiological and hormone-supporting condition you can be in) so that you can keep your weight off and continue to live life in great shape.

Pursue Good Stress Management

We women are often the caretakers of children, elderly parents, and other family members, and we often do not take the time to care for ourselves. Stress is prevalent, and stress can be an incredible enemy to our health and happiness.

If we are chronically under stress, our body produces very high amounts of cortisol. Eventually the adrenal glands burn out and we wind up releasing too little cortisol, which in turn causes a decrease in progesterone and oxytocin. This results in feelings of disconnection, a sense of burnout, and inflammation.

Eating and living alkaline is a big part of the solution. This not only helps restore cortisol to healthy levels but also helps reset our daily circadian rhythm, boosts mood, decreases joint pain, promotes better sleeping habits, and helps shed pounds.

Improving your stress management helps move your body into a state of being more net alkaline, instead of more net acidic. Identify ways to control stress—find the methods that work for you. And learn to manage your thoughts around the stress you simply can't control. Stress is a normal part of life, and it can even be healthy when we perceive that we have control over it and can find internal peace within it. Many of my Clean 16 strategies in Chapter 10 can help you manage stress better.

Avoid Obesogens

Obesogens are artificial chemicals believed to contribute to obesity. They are found in various food containers, baby bottles, toys, plastics, cookware, and especially skincare products. Obesogens are a category of endocrine disruptors—chemicals that can interfere with your hormones. When these chemicals enter your body, they can disrupt its normal hormone function and promote fat gain.

Some endocrine disruptors exert their effects by stimulating estrogen receptors on cells so that these substances can enter cells and cause harmful effects in both women and men. Estrogen receptors have been described as "promiscuous," meaning that they will latch on to anything that looks even remotely like an estrogen.

Some of the most common hormone disruptors are parabens, found in thousands of cosmetics and other products, and phthalates, present in fragrances. Other harmful additives in skincare products are sodium lauryl sulfate and sodium laureth sulfate, which are often contaminated with carcinogens, and petroleum, which is also tinged with cancer-causing agents.

It's best to switch to natural/organic cosmetics and grooming products and use olive oil or goat's milk soaps. Or try making your own cosmetics and skincare products from natural sources. It's easy to do, and there are many recipes on the Internet.

Get Quality Sleep

If you have trouble sleeping, your body will be more acidic. So naturally you'll want to take action to pursue restorative sleep. My Keto-Green protocol balances blood sugar levels and optimizes hormones, improving sleep and helping to reset your circadian rhythm. It is also an alkaline diet, which is known to promote restful sleep. Creating a lovely, clutter-free environment in your bedroom and turning off sleep-disrupting electronics prior to bedtime is important as well.

Create Positivity

Negative thinking isn't just bad for your mood; it's also bad for your brain and your hormone balance. Chronic anger, hate, and resentment produce stress, causing your adrenals to release too much cortisol. Over time, high levels of cortisol shrink the hippocampus (the brain area associated with memory and emotions) and can cause more negative thinking.

I understand that you can't always remove stressors from your life. But maybe you can change your perceptions and responses to some of them. As Dale Carnegie wrote in his bestseller *How to Win Friends and Influence People:* "Everybody in the world is seeking happiness—and there is one sure way to find it. That is by controlling your thoughts. Happiness doesn't depend on outward conditions. It depends on inner conditions."

Put More Oxytocin in Your Life

This amazing hormone will nourish your soul and your relationships—and it's easy to boost it. Laugh, play, hug, look into someone's eyes and smile, give gratitude and thanks, play with a pet, and stay in the present (so difficult for many of us). So yes, you can love that belly fat away!

Make a proactive effort to carve out time in each day to connect with others—in person and not just on social media. Connecting to others in positive ways is very good medicine.

Exercise! Even better, exercise in a group or club team, just like when we were in school.

Remember that the "O" in oxytocin also is the "O" in orgasm! Making love and staying intimate is a great way to flood your body with oxytocin, which then counters cortisol's negative effects.

You must put yourself first and continue living the full Keto-Green lifestyle. Along with it, love yourself, love your life, and pursue the quality of life you want to have. I want a long, happy, healthy, prosperous, amazing life, filled with good friendships, and I want you to have this too.

APPENDIX A

The Keto-Green 16 Recipes

BEVERAGES, SMOOTHIES, AND BROTHS

KETO COFFEE OR TEA

(Vegan friendly without the egg and collagen)

SERVES 1

1 cup brewed coffee or tea
1 tablespoon coconut oil or MCT oil
1 teaspoon coconut ghee

OPTIONAL ADDITIONS:
   1 egg yolk (leave out if vegan)
   1 teaspoon to 1 tablespoon collagen powder (leave out if
   vegan)
   ¼ teaspoon cinnamon and/or cardamom
   1 to 5 drops liquid stevia, or liquid monkfruit or pure
   vanilla extract

Place all ingredients in a blender and blend until smooth.

Note: If you're concerned about the potential risk of salmonella in raw egg yolks, you can make them safe by using pasteurized eggs. To pasteurize eggs at home, simply pour enough water in a saucepan to cover the eggs. Heat the water to 140 degrees. Using a spoon, slowly lower the eggs into the water. Keep the eggs in the water for about 3 minutes. This should be enough to kill any potential bacteria without cooking the eggs. Remove the eggs from the water, let cool, and store in the fridge for 6–8 weeks.

DR. ANNA'S BASIC KETO-GREEN SHAKE

(Vegan friendly)

MAKES 1 SERVING

*1 scoop Dr. Anna Cabeca's Keto-Alkaline Protein Shake
or Dr. Anna Cabeca Keto-Green Meal Replacement or
similar product (see note)
1 tablespoon MCT or coconut oil
2 scoops Dr. Anna Cabeca Mighty Maca Plus
8 ounces water*

Place all ingredients in a blender and blend until smooth.

Note: You can substitute my Keto-Green or Keto-Alkaline Protein
powders with a similar one you love and do well with. Just be conscientious about keeping the macronutrient and micronutrient profiles close.

DR. ANNA'S FAVORITE
SUPER KETO-GREEN SHAKE

(Vegan friendly)

MAKES 1 SERVING

1 scoop Dr. Anna Cabeca Keto-Green Meal Replacement
*   or similar product (see note)*
1 tablespoon MCT or coconut oil
2 scoops Dr. Anna Cabeca Mighty Maca Plus
1 handful kale
1 stalk celery
½-inch-thick slice fresh ginger
¼ avocado
Dash cardamom or a few leaves of fresh mint
1 teaspoon chia seeds, ground flaxseeds, hulled pumpkin
*   seeds, or hulled sunflower seeds*
8 ounces water
3 or 4 ice cubes

Place all ingredients in a blender and blend until smooth.

Note: You can substitute my Keto-Green Meal Replacement with a similar product you love and do well with. Just be conscientious about keeping the macronutrient and micronutrient profiles close.

Variations: With any of my Keto-Green shakes or smoothies, add in one or a few great-tasting alkaline additions listed here. Mix and match to come up with your own delicious recipes.

Fresh ginger	*Cilantro*	*Cinnamon*
Avocado	*Collagen powder*	*Cardamom*
Kale, spinach,	*Coconut water,*	*Pure vanilla extract*
and/or other	*coconut milk, or*	
greens	*unsweetened coconut*	
Mint	*flakes*	

PINEAPPLE KETO-GREEN SMOOTHIE

(Vegan friendly)

SERVES 2

2 cups unsweetened almond or coconut milk
½ teaspoon ground turmeric
2 teaspoons ground flaxseeds
2 teaspoons chia seeds
1 avocado
2 tablespoons MCT oil
Juice of 1 small lemon
1 cup frozen pineapple, mango, or papaya
⅔ cup frozen cauliflower rice (see note)
4 or 5 ice cubes
2 scoops Dr. Anna Cabeca Keto-Green Meal Replacement
  or similar product

Place all ingredients except Keto-Green powder in a blender and blend until smooth.

Add protein powder and blend until combined. If the smoothie is too thick, add filtered water until you reach the desired consistency.

Serve cold and store leftovers in the fridge.

HOW TO "RICE" CAULIFLOWER

You can make your own cauliflower rice. Trim ½ head cauliflower and cut into florets. Lightly steam the cauliflower, then place in a food processor and pulse until it becomes the texture of rice. Freeze it for use in this recipe.

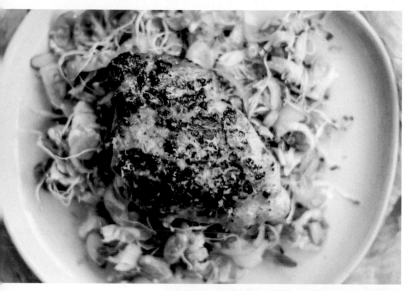

Lemon Pepper Chicken with Brussels Sprouts Slaw (page 235)

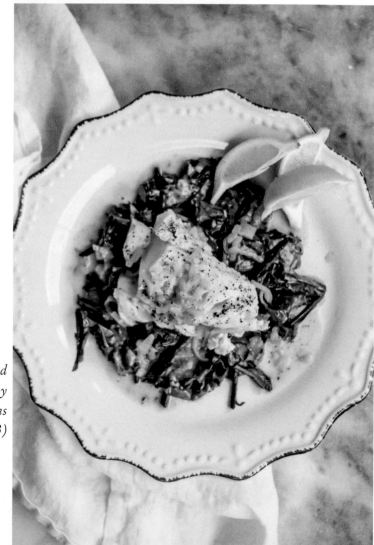

Lemon Poached Fish with Garlicky Beet Greens (page 263)

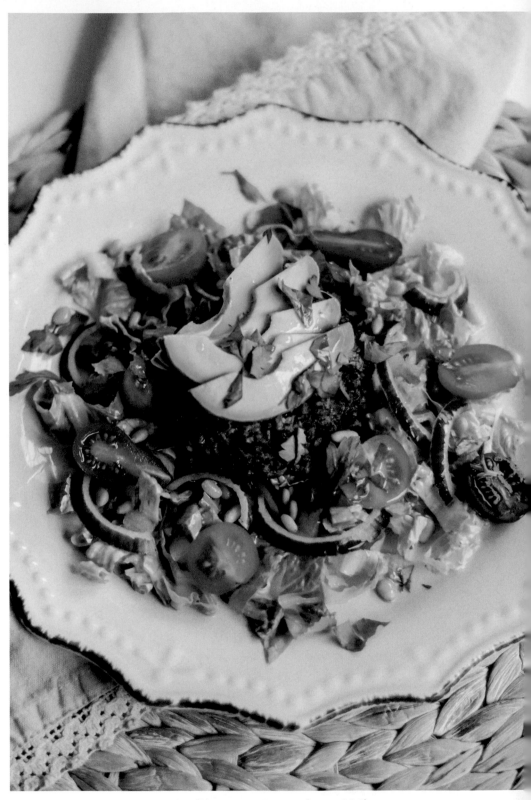

Mediterranean Burger (page 231)

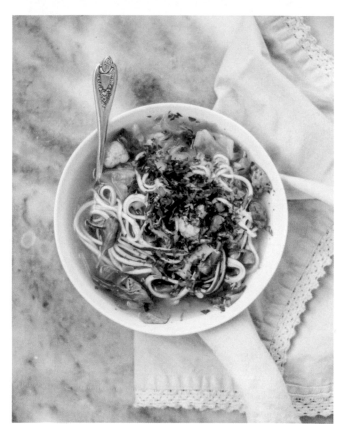

Not Your Mama's Cabbage Soup (page 261)

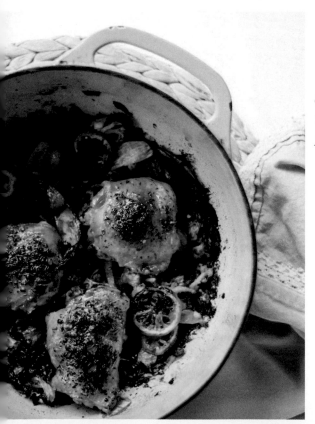

One-Pot Roasted Chicken and Veggies with Caramelized Lemons (page 258)

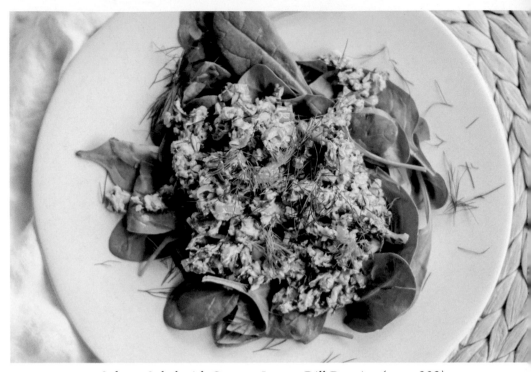

Salmon Salad with Creamy Lemon Dill Dressing (page 232)

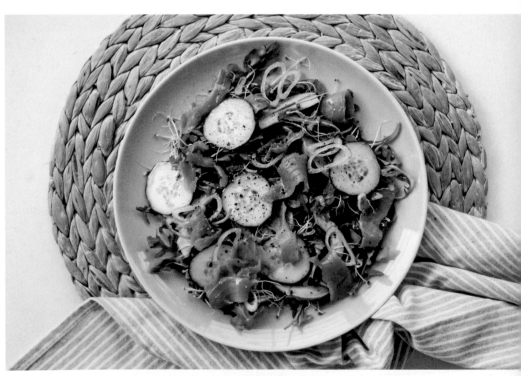

Smoked Salmon and Avocado Salad (page 222)

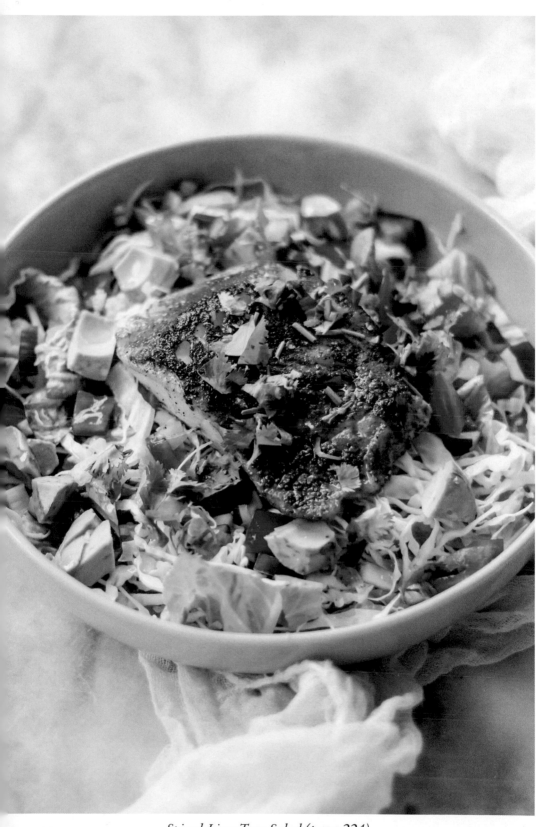

Spiced Lime Taco Salad (page 224)

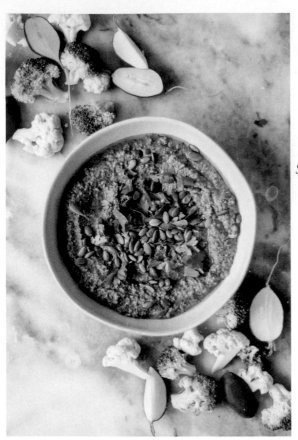

Spicy Pumpkin Seed Dip (page 281)

Turmeric Meatballs with Parsley and Sprouts Slaw (page 266)

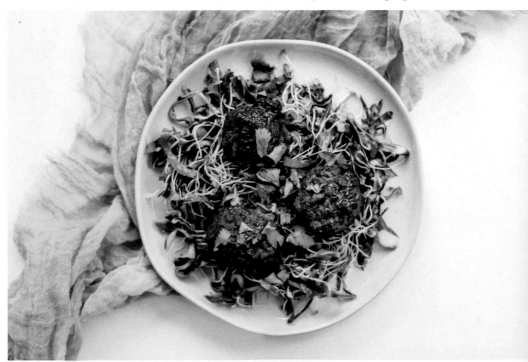

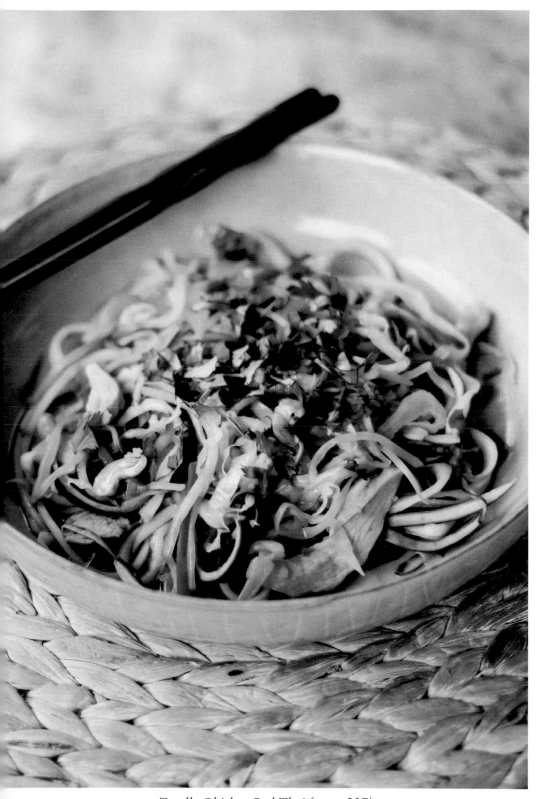

Zoodle Chicken Pad Thai (page 237)

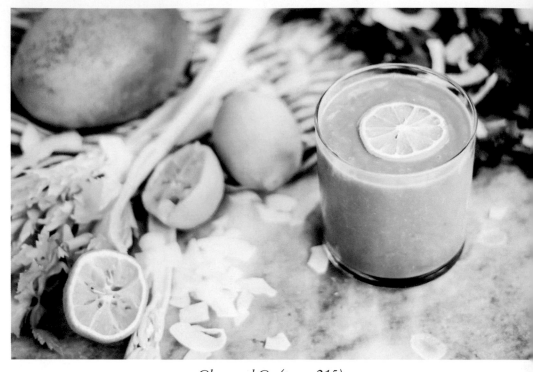

Glow and Go (page 215)

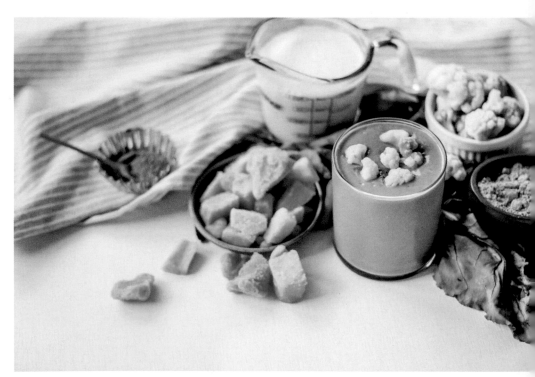

Strength Builder (page 217)

CHOCOLATE KETO-GREEN SMOOTHIE

(Vegan friendly)

SERVES 2

2 cups unsweetened almond or coconut milk
2 teaspoons ground flaxseeds
2 teaspoons chia seeds
1 avocado
⅔ cup full-fat coconut milk
4 cups spinach or other dark leafy greens
Pinch sea salt
4 to 5 ice cubes
2 scoops Dr. Anna Cabeca Mighty Maca Plus (see note)
2 scoops Dr. Anna Cabeca Keto-Green Meal Replacement
  or similar product (see note)

Place all ingredients except protein powder in a blender and blend until smooth.

Add protein powder and blend until combined. If the smoothie is too thick, add filtered water until you reach the desired consistency.

Serve cold and store leftovers in the fridge until ready to enjoy.

Note: To substitute for the Keto-Green Chocolate Meal Replacement and Mighty Maca Plus powders, replace them with ¼ cup almond butter, 1 tablespoon cocoa powder, 1 handful kale, and 1 handful broccoli sprouts.

WILLPOWER MAMA

(Vegan friendly)

SERVES 2

2½ cups unsweetened almond milk
1 tablespoon MCT oil
1 cup frozen avocado chunks
½ cup sprouts
2 cups frozen kale
1½ teaspoons cinnamon
½ teaspoon cardamom

Combine all ingredients in a blender and blend until smooth.

FAT BURNER

....

(Vegan friendly)

SERVES 2

2½ cups unsweetened coconut milk
2 cups frozen spinach
1 cup frozen avocado chunks
½ cup frozen pineapple
½ cup frozen papaya

Combine all ingredients in a blender and blend until smooth.

SEXY SMOOTHIE

SERVES 2

2½ cups unsweetened cashew milk
2 cups frozen cauliflower florets
2 scoops protein powder
2 scoops collagen powder (available at pharmacies and
   health food stores)
1 tablespoon MCT oil
2 teaspoons cacao nibs
1 teaspoon cinnamon
¼ teaspoon cayenne pepper

Combine all ingredients in a blender and blend until smooth.

AGELESS BEAUTY

SERVES 2

2½ cups unsweetened coconut water
½ cup frozen mango
2 cups frozen kale
2 scoops collagen powder (available at pharmacies and
  health food stores)
2 teaspoons ground turmeric

Combine all ingredients in a blender and blend until smooth.

MUSCLE MAVEN

(Vegan friendly)

SERVES 2

2½ cups unsweetened coconut milk
2 tablespoons almond butter
1 tablespoon MCT oil
2 scoops Dr. Anna Cabeca Keto-Green Meal Replacement
   or similar product
2 cups sprouts
½ cup unsweetened coconut flakes

Combine all ingredients in a blender and blend until smooth.

CLEAN AND PURE

(Vegan friendly)

SERVES 2

2½ cups unsweetened coconut water
1 medium cucumber
2 stalks celery
1 cup parsley
1 cup frozen avocado chunks
Juice and zest of 1 lemon
1 tablespoon grated fresh ginger

Combine all ingredients in a blender and blend until smooth.

POWER UP SHAKE

SERVES 2

2½ cups water or unsweetened coconut water

2 scoops Dr. Anna Cabeca Keto-Green Meal Replacement
   or similar product

2 scoops Dr. Anna Cabeca Mighty Maca Plus or plain
   maca

3 tablespoons MCT oil

2 scoops collagen powder

2 tablespoons grated fresh ginger

½ cup clover sprouts

1½ cups spinach

1 cup arugula

6 pili nuts

2 beet greens leaves (no stems)

Combine all ingredients in a blender and blend until smooth.

GLOW AND GO

(Vegan friendly)

SERVES 2

2½ cups unsweetened coconut water
2 cups frozen kale
1 cup frozen avocado chunks
Juice and zest of 1 lemon
2 stalks celery
½ cup unsweetened coconut flakes
½ cup frozen mango

Combine all ingredients in a blender and blend until smooth.

DETOXIFIER

(Vegan friendly)

SERVES 2

2½ cups unsweetened coconut water
¼ cup coconut water kefir
2 stalks celery
Juice and zest of 1 lemon
1 cup frozen kale
1 cup frozen spinach
½ cup frozen pineapple

Combine all ingredients in a blender and blend until smooth.

STRENGTH BUILDER

(Vegan friendly)

SERVES 2

2½ cups unsweetened almond milk
2 scoops Dr. Anna Cabeca Keto-Green Meal Replacement or similar product
2 scoops Dr. Anna Cabeca Mighty Maca Plus or plain maca
2 cups beet greens (no stems) or kale
1 cup frozen cauliflower florets
½ cup frozen mango

Combine all ingredients in a blender and blend until smooth.

TROPICAL TURMERIC MILKSHAKE

(Vegan friendly)

SERVES 2

⅓ *cup frozen mango*
⅓ *cup frozen papaya*
1 *cup full-fat coconut milk*
2 *teaspoons lemon juice*
1 *tablespoon grated fresh ginger*
1½ *teaspoons ground turmeric*

Combine all ingredients in a blender and blend until smooth.

DR. ANNA'S KOOL KETO MOCKTAIL

(Vegan friendly)

MAKES 1 SERVING

Fresh mint, 2 to 3 leaves
Juice of 1 lime or lemon
Ice to fill glass
Sparkling water to fill glass
Pomegranate seeds (optional)

In a large glass, muddle together mint and lime or lemon.
   Add ice and sparkling water.
   For added color, add pomegranate seeds.

KETO BONE BROTH

MAKES 1 GALLON

2 carrots, roughly chopped
2 stalks celery, including leafy part, roughly chopped
1 medium onion, roughly chopped
7 cloves garlic, peeled and smashed
3½ pounds bones from grass-fed beef (preferably joints
  and knuckles)
2 bay leaves
2 teaspoons sea salt
2 tablespoons apple cider vinegar

Place all the ingredients into a slow cooker. Add water to cover by 1 inch. Cook for 8 to 10 hours on low.

Use a shallow spoon to carefully skim any scum off the top of the broth. Pour the broth through a fine strainer and discard the solids. Taste the broth and add salt as needed. Store in a glass container. The broth will keep for 3 days in the fridge and 3 months in the freezer.

Variations: Feel free to substitute chicken, fish, or pork bones or to combine them all. Also, try adding dried mushrooms or 2 tablespoons fish sauce in place of the salt to dramatically boost the flavor of the broth.

KETO ALKALINE BROTH

(Vegan friendly)

MAKES ABOUT 1 GALLON BROTH

2 carrots, roughly chopped
2 onions, roughly chopped
4 cloves garlic, smashed
½ head cabbage, roughly chopped
1 bunch celery, roughly chopped
1-inch piece ginger root, sliced
½ bunch parsley
1 8-inch strip kombu seaweed
2 bay leaves
1 teaspoon black peppercorns
1 tablespoon sea salt

Place all ingredients in a soup pot, add water to cover by 1 inch, and bring to a boil. Reduce heat and simmer for 2 to 4 hours. Adjust the salt.

Strain the broth, cool, and store in glass containers in the fridge for 3 to 4 days or in the freezer for up to 6 months.

LUNCHES

SMOKED SALMON AND AVOCADO SALAD

SERVES 2

SALAD

4 cups arugula
1 avocado, sliced
1 small shallot, sliced
1 cup sprouts
1 cup sliced cucumber
8 to 10 ounces smoked salmon

DRESSING

¼ cup olive oil
⅓ cup lemon juice
Zest of 1 lemon
1 clove garlic, grated
Sea salt
Freshly ground black pepper

In a large bowl, combine all ingredients for salad.

In a small bowl, whisk together oil, lemon juice, lemon zest, and garlic. Season with salt and pepper. Drizzle over salad and toss.

KOREAN BEEF AND CABBAGE

SERVES 2

2 tablespoons coconut oil
4 cloves garlic, minced
2 tablespoons grated fresh ginger
1 tablespoon chili paste
8 ounces ground beef
3 cups shredded cabbage
4 scallions, cut lengthwise into 8 pieces
3 tablespoons coconut aminos
2 tablespoons lime juice
1 teaspoon sea salt
1 teaspoon freshly ground black pepper
1 handful fresh basil leaves
1 handful fresh mint leaves
1 handful fresh cilantro leaves

Heat coconut oil in a large skillet over medium-high heat. Add garlic, ginger, and chili paste. Cook for about 1 minute, until fragrant.

Add beef and cook for about 3 minutes, or until beef is nearly done. Add cabbage, scallions, coconut aminos, and lime juice. Season with salt and pepper. Cook for another 5 minutes, or until cabbage is tender.

Top with basil, mint, and cilantro.

SPICED LIME TACO SALAD

SERVES 2

SALAD

½ teaspoon sea salt
½ teaspoon freshly ground black pepper
½ teaspoon cumin
½ teaspoon chili powder
¼ teaspoon paprika
8 ounces cod or other firm white fish
2 tablespoons coconut oil
1 head romaine lettuce, chopped
1 cup shredded cabbage
½ small red onion, chopped
1 medium vine-ripened tomato, chopped
1 avocado, cubed

DRESSING

3 tablespoons olive oil
¼ cup lime juice
Zest of 1 lime
Sea salt

In a small bowl, combine salt, pepper, cumin, chili powder, and paprika. Season all sides of the fish with the spice mixture.

Heat coconut oil in a medium skillet over medium-high heat. Add fish and cook for 3 to 4 minutes per side, or until cooked through and fish flakes easily with fork. Set aside.

In a large bowl, combine lettuce, cabbage, onion, tomato, and avocado.

In a small bowl, whisk together oil, lime juice, and lime zest. Season with salt. Drizzle over salad and toss. Top with a serving of fish.

FARMER'S MARKET BOWL

SERVES 2

3 tablespoons olive oil, divided
¼ cup lemon juice
3 cloves garlic, minced
1 cup halved Brussels sprouts
1 cup cauliflower florets
1 cup broccoli florets
8 ounces skinless, boneless chicken thighs
Sea salt
Freshly ground black pepper
1 zucchini, spiralized
2 cups spinach
1 handful parsley
1 lemon, cut into wedges

Preheat oven to 400 degrees.

In a large bowl, whisk together 2 tablespoons oil, lemon juice, and garlic. Add Brussels sprouts, cauliflower, and broccoli and toss well. Transfer to a parchment-lined rimmed baking sheet.

Place chicken on baking sheet next to veggies and brush with remaining 1 tablespoon oil. Season chicken and veggies with salt and pepper. Roast for 30 minutes or until chicken is cooked through and veggies are tender.

While chicken and veggies cook, prep the zucchini noodles. Bring a medium pot of water to a boil, add zucchini, and cook for 30 seconds to 1 minute. Drain, then rinse and set aside.

Once chicken and veggies are ready, assemble the bowls. Start with a base of zucchini noodles, then add 1 cup spinach, a serving of chicken and roasted veggies, and finish with a garnish of parsley and a lemon wedge or two. If there are any cooking juices in the bottom of the baking sheet, drizzle them on top of each bowl.

SKILLET GARLIC CHICKEN AND GREENS

SERVES 2

3 tablespoons ghee, divided
4 cloves garlic, minced
1 teaspoon sea salt, divided
½ teaspoon lemon pepper
8 to 10 ounces skinless, boneless chicken breast
1 tablespoon apple cider vinegar
4 cups spinach

Melt 2 tablespoons of the ghee. In a small bowl, combine melted ghee, garlic, ½ teaspoon salt, and lemon pepper. Using your hands, rub mixture all over chicken.

Heat a medium skillet over medium-high heat. If there is any garlic-ghee mixture left, add it to the skillet; if not, add a teaspoon or two of additional ghee. Then add chicken. Cook for 5 to 6 minutes per side or until cooked through. Once done, remove from pan and turn heat down to medium low.

Add the remaining 1 tablespoon ghee and the apple cider vinegar to the skillet. Add spinach, season with remaining salt, and cook for about 3 minutes, or until spinach is completely wilted. Serve with chicken.

KETO-GREEN CRUDITÉS
WITH CHIPOTLE CASHEW DIP

SERVES 2

CASHEW DIP

½ cup raw cashews, soaked in water for at least 2 hours
2 cloves garlic
2 tablespoons olive oil
1 chipotle pepper in adobo sauce
1 tablespoon lime juice
2 tablespoons water
½ teaspoon sea salt

VEGGIES

3 cups raw veggies (any approved for Keto-Green
16—cucumber, cauliflower, broccoli, avocado, etc.)

PROTEIN

8 ounces smoked salmon

In a food processor, combine all ingredients for cashew dip. Process until smooth. Serve with veggies on the side and a serving of smoked salmon.

30-MINUTE KETO-GREEN SOUP

. . . .

SERVES 2

2 tablespoons ghee
1 medium onion, chopped
2 stalks celery, chopped
2 tablespoons grated fresh ginger
3 cloves garlic, minced
5 cups bone broth or low-sodium chicken broth
2 cups halved Brussels sprouts
1 cup cauliflower florets
Sea salt
Freshly ground black pepper
8 ounces cooked protein of your choice (chicken, fish,
  tofu, tempeh, beef, etc.)
2 scallions, chopped
1 handful cilantro, chopped
1 handful parsley, chopped

Heat ghee in a large pot over medium-high heat. Add onion, celery, ginger, and garlic. Cook for about 2 minutes or until onion is slightly tender. Add broth, Brussels sprouts, and cauliflower, and season with salt and pepper.

Bring to a boil, then reduce heat to medium low and cook for about 20 minutes or until veggies are fork tender. Stir in protein and heat through. Top with scallions, cilantro, and parsley.

CRUNCHY SUMMER SLAW WITH HALIBUT

SERVES 2

SLAW

2 stalks celery, chopped
2 cups thinly sliced purple cabbage
1 cup sprouts
3 large radishes, sliced
½ onion, sliced
3 tablespoons MCT oil
¼ cup lemon juice
1 tablespoon grated fresh ginger
1 clove garlic, minced
Sea salt
Freshly ground black pepper

HALIBUT

½ teaspoon sea salt
½ teaspoon lemon pepper
¼ teaspoon garlic powder
¼ teaspoon paprika
8 ounces halibut filets or other firm-fleshed white fish
2 tablespoons coconut oil

In a large bowl, combine celery, cabbage, sprouts, radishes, and onion. In a small bowl, whisk together MCT oil, lemon juice, ginger, and garlic; season with salt and pepper. Drizzle over veggies, toss to combine, and set the slaw aside.

In a small bowl, mix together salt, lemon pepper, garlic powder, and paprika. Pat fish dry and season with spice mixture.

Heat coconut oil in a skillet over medium-high heat. Add halibut and cook for 3 to 4 minutes per side, or until fish flakes easily with fork.

Serve fish with a generous helping of slaw.

GOLDEN CHICKEN THAI SALAD

SERVES 2

8 ounces cooked chicken
1 shallot, chopped
1 stalk celery, chopped
1 cup chopped cilantro
1 avocado, cubed
¼ cup sliced almonds
2 cloves garlic, minced
2 teaspoons grated fresh ginger
1 teaspoon ground turmeric
½ teaspoon sea salt
½ teaspoon freshly ground black pepper
½ teaspoon cumin
¼ cup lime juice
⅓ cup full-fat coconut milk
4 radicchio leaves (or lettuce)

In a large bowl, combine all ingredients except radicchio. Serve in radicchio leaves.

MEDITERRANEAN BURGER

SERVES 2

BURGERS

8 to 10 ounces ground beef
2 tablespoons olive oil
1 egg
½ red onion, finely chopped
3 cloves garlic, minced
½ cup chopped parsley
1 teaspoon sea salt
1 teaspoon freshly ground black pepper

SALAD

1 head romaine lettuce, chopped
1 cup chopped heirloom or cherry tomatoes
½ red onion, sliced
1 avocado, sliced
2 tablespoons pine nuts

DRESSING

3 tablespoons olive oil
¼ cup lemon juice
Sea salt
Freshly ground black pepper

Preheat an outdoor or indoor grill to medium-high heat.

In a large bowl, combine all ingredients for burgers. Mix well with hands and divide into two patties.

Grease grill grate and cook burgers for 3 to 5 minutes per side, or until done to your liking. Remove from grill and let rest for 5 minutes while you prepare salad.

In a large bowl, combine lettuce, tomatoes, onion, avocado, and pine nuts. In a separate small bowl, whisk together oil and lemon juice, and season with salt and pepper. Dress salad with vinaigrette, toss, and serve with burger patty on top.

SALMON SALAD
WITH CREAMY LEMON DILL DRESSING

SERVES 2

DRESSING

¼ cup lemon juice
Zest of 1 lemon
½ cup chopped fresh dill
4 tablespoons MCT oil
½ teaspoon sea salt

SALAD

8 ounces canned or poached salmon, drained
1 stalk celery, chopped
3 scallions, chopped
1 cup chopped parsley
4 cups spinach, romaine, kale, or other leafy greens

In a blender, combine all ingredients for dressing. Blend until smooth and creamy-looking.

In a large bowl, combine salmon, celery, scallions, and parsley. Add dressing and toss well. Adjust seasoning.

Serve salmon mixture over the greens.

BEEF AND CRUCIFEROUS TACOS WITH AVOCADO LIME CREMA

SERVES 2

CREMA

1 avocado, cubed
¼ cup lime juice
½ jalapeño, seeded and chopped
1 cup chopped cilantro
⅓ cup full-fat coconut milk
½ teaspoon sea salt

TACOS

2 tablespoons olive oil
8 ounces ground beef
1 small onion, chopped
3 cloves garlic, minced
1 cup chopped broccoli florets
1 cup chopped cauliflower florets
½ cup shaved Brussels sprouts
1 teaspoon sea salt
1 teaspoon freshly ground black pepper
1 teaspoon cumin
1 teaspoon chili powder
½ teaspoon cayenne pepper
½ teaspoon paprika
4 cabbage leaves
1 handful cilantro, chopped
1 handful sprouts

In a blender, combine all ingredients for crema. Blend until smooth and set aside.

Heat olive oil in a large skillet over medium-high heat. Add beef and cook for 3 minutes, or until browned. Pour off any fat in the pan. Add onion, garlic, broccoli, cauliflower, and

Brussels sprouts. Add salt, pepper, cumin, chili powder, cayenne, and paprika. Cook, stirring regularly, for another 6 to 7 minutes, or until veggies are fork-tender.

Serve beef mixture inside cabbage "tacos" and top with crema, cilantro, and sprouts.

LEMON PEPPER CHICKEN
WITH BRUSSELS SPROUTS SLAW

. . . .

SERVES 2

SLAW

2 cups shaved Brussels sprouts
1 cup sprouts
1 shallot, sliced thin
⅓ cup sliced almonds
¼ cup lemon juice
2 tablespoons olive oil
Sea salt
Freshly ground black pepper

CHICKEN

2 tablespoons lemon juice
2 teaspoons lemon zest
4 cloves garlic, minced
¾ teaspoon sea salt
1 teaspoon freshly ground black pepper
8 ounces skinless, boneless chicken thighs
2 tablespoons ghee

In a large bowl, combine Brussels sprouts, sprouts, shallot, almonds, lemon juice, and olive oil. Season with salt and pepper. Cover and set aside.

In a small bowl, mix together lemon juice, zest, garlic, salt, and pepper to create a paste. Rub on both sides of the chicken.

Heat ghee in a medium skillet over medium-high heat. Cook chicken for 4 to 5 minutes per side, or until cooked through.

Serve chicken with a heap of slaw.

ROASTED CABBAGE
WITH CHICKEN AND SHALLOTS

SERVES 2

1 head cabbage, cut into wedges
2 shallots, chopped
8 to 10 ounces bone-in chicken thighs
4 cloves garlic, minced
Juice of 1 large lemon
3 tablespoons ghee, melted
1 teaspoon sea salt
1 teaspoon freshly ground black pepper
¼ cup sliced almonds, toasted

Preheat oven to 400 degrees.

In a baking dish or Dutch oven, arrange cabbage, shallots, and chicken. In a small bowl, whisk together garlic, lemon juice, and ghee. Pour evenly over chicken and veggies. Season everything with salt and pepper.

Place in oven and roast for 30 to 40 minutes, or until cabbage is tender and chicken is cooked through.

Serve with toasted almonds on top.

Tip: Save bones for bone broth!

ZOODLE CHICKEN PAD THAI

. . . .

SERVES 2

2 tablespoons coconut oil
3 cloves garlic, minced
2 tablespoons grated fresh ginger
1 small onion, sliced
1 red chile (or jalapeño), seeded and chopped
¼ cup chicken broth
8 ounces skinless, boneless chicken breast, cut into thin
  strips
½ cup shredded carrot
1 cup bean sprouts
1 cup chopped cabbage
2 scallions, sliced lengthwise into 4 pieces
1 large zucchini, spiralized
¼ cup cashews
¼ cup coconut aminos
Juice of 2 large limes
1 teaspoon sea salt
½ teaspoon freshly ground black pepper
1 handful cilantro, chopped

Heat coconut oil in a large wok or non-stick skillet over medium-high heat. Add garlic, ginger, onion, and chile and cook for 2 to 3 minutes.

Add broth and chicken, stir, and cook for 3 more minutes. Add carrot, bean sprouts, cabbage, and scallions. Cook for about 4 minutes, or until veggies are tender.

Add zucchini, cashews, coconut aminos, lime juice, salt, and pepper. Cook for another 2 minutes or just until zucchini is heated through. Serve with cilantro on top.

EGG HAND SALAD

SERVES 2

4 hard-boiled eggs, peeled and chopped
2 stalks celery, chopped
3 scallions, chopped
1 avocado, cubed
½ cup chopped parsley
½ cup chopped cilantro
⅓ cup plain coconut yogurt
Juice and zest of 1 lemon
2 teaspoons Dijon mustard
1 teaspoon sea salt
1 teaspoon freshly ground black pepper
¼ teaspoon paprika
4 leaves romaine or butter lettuce

In a large bowl, combine all ingredients except lettuce. Toss gently. Serve in lettuce leaves.

CURRIED CABBAGE KETO-GREEN SOUP

(Vegan friendly)

SERVES 2

2 tablespoons coconut ghee
½ cup chopped onion
2 celery stalks, diced
2 cups shredded cabbage
2 cups Keto Alkaline Broth (page 221)
½ to 1 teaspoon curry powder
½ teaspoon cayenne pepper
2 cups fresh spinach or baby kale
Juice of ½ lime or lemon
1 cup canned black soybeans, drained
2 tablespoons extra-virgin olive oil
¼ cup chopped cilantro or parsley
½ cup kimchi

Heat ghee over medium-high heat in a soup pot. Add onion, celery, and cabbage and sauté 5 minutes.

Lower heat. Add broth, curry powder, and cayenne. Stir in spinach and cook until wilted, about 2 minutes.

Add lime or lemon juice and beans and stir to combine. Cook on low about 5 to 10 minutes, until flavors blend.

Place mixture in a large soup bowl, drizzle with olive oil, and garnish with fresh herbs. Adjust the seasonings. Serve with kimchi on the side.

KETO-GREEN GAZPACHO

(Vegan friendly)

SERVES 2

2 tablespoons chopped white onion
1 clove garlic
½ jalapeño, seeded and chopped
2 cups fresh spinach
½ cup cilantro
½ medium cucumber
1 avocado
¼ teaspoon sea salt
Juice of 1 lime
2 cups Keto Alkaline Broth (page 221)
½ cup ice cubes
2 tablespoons extra-virgin olive oil
2 tablespoons hemp seeds

Place all ingredients except for the olive oil and hemp seeds in a blender and blend until smooth. If too thick, add water to achieve desired texture. Pour into bowls.

Drizzle with olive oil and top with hemp seeds. Serve cold.

Store leftovers in a glass container in the refrigerator for up to 3 days.

KETO-GREEN PÂTÉ
ENDIVE BOATS

. . . .

(Vegan friendly)

SERVES 2

1 tablespoon coconut ghee
¼ yellow onion, chopped
1 cup shiitake mushrooms
2 cloves garlic, minced
¼ cup walnuts
¼ cup macadamia nuts
1 tablespoon nutritional yeast
¼ cup chopped parsley
1 teaspoon dried rosemary or thyme
Juice of ¼ lemon
Sea salt
Freshly ground black pepper
1 medium head Belgian endive
Extra-virgin olive oil

Warm the ghee over medium heat in a skillet. Sauté the onion for about 3 minutes or until softened. Add the mushrooms and cook for another 3 minutes. If the mixture seems dry, add a little water, about 1 tablespoon at a time. Stir in the garlic and cook until aromatic, about 1 to 2 minutes. Remove from heat.

Place the walnuts, macadamia nuts, nutritional yeast, parsley, rosemary, and lemon juice in a food processor and pulse until chunky. Season with salt and pepper.

Add the mushroom mixture to the blender and blend until smooth. If the mixture seems dry, add a little water or broth, about 1 tablespoon at a time. Adjust seasoning.

Slice root end off endive, then separate into leaves to make "boats."

Spoon 2 tablespoons pâté onto the white end of each endive leaf. Drizzle with olive oil.

The pâté can be prepared in advance and stored in a glass container in the refrigerator for up to 3 days.

YOGURT BOWL WITH KETO-GREEN-OLA

(Vegan friendly)

SERVES 2

2 containers (150 g each) plain Kite Hill dairy-free
yogurt or unsweetened coconut yogurt
2 scoops Dr. Anna Cabeca's Keto-Alkaline Protein Shake
2 teaspoons MCT oil
2 tablespoons chopped pecans
2 tablespoons unsweetened shredded coconut
1 tablespoon cacao
¼ cup chopped pineapple, mango, or papaya

Place yogurt in 2 bowls. In each bowl, mix in 1 scoop protein powder and 1 teaspoon MCT oil.

Top one side of each bowl with pecans, coconut, and nibs and then arrange fruit on the other side. Serve immediately.

TOASTED TEMPEH NOODLE BOWL WITH CILANTRO LIME GREENS

(Vegan friendly)

SERVES 2

2 tablespoons coconut oil, divided
1 package (4 ounces) tempeh, cut into ¼-inch cubes
¼ teaspoon sea salt, divided
Freshly ground black pepper, to taste
½ bunch watercress (about 3 ounces), trimmed and
   chopped
2 cups trimmed and chopped bok choy
1 7-ounce package Wonder Noodles (shirataki noodles)
   cooked as directed
1½ teaspoons gluten-free tamari
1 teaspoon fish sauce (optional—leave off if vegan)
½ cup chopped cilantro
1½ teaspoons sesame oil
Juice of ½ lime
2 tablespoons coarsely chopped raw almonds or cashews
½ avocado, cubed

Heat 1 tablespoon coconut oil over medium-high heat in a skillet. Brown the tempeh for about 3 minutes on each side, until slightly golden and toasted. Season with sea salt and pepper and set aside.

Add remaining coconut oil to the pan. Stir in the watercress and bok choy and cook until just wilted, about 2 to 3 minutes. Season with remaining salt.

Stir in the Wonder Noodles and lower heat. Add in tempeh. Cook for another 3 minutes to allow flavors to combine. Remove from heat and then stir in the tamari, fish sauce (if using), cilantro, sesame oil, and lime juice.

Evenly divide the vegetable mixture between 2 bowls. Top each bowl with 1 tablespoon chopped almonds and half of the avocado.

Store any leftovers in the refrigerator in a glass container for up to 5 days.

KETO-GREEN RAW WRAPS WITH ZUCCHINI-WHITE BEAN HUMMUS

(Vegan friendly)

SERVES 2

8 collard leaves
¼ medium zucchini, chopped
¼ cup canned white kidney beans, drained
¼ avocado
2 tablespoons chopped onion
1 clove garlic
2 tablespoons hemp seeds
1 tablespoon chopped parsley
1½ tablespoons apple cider vinegar
1½ tablespoons gluten-free tamari
1 tablespoon nutritional yeast
⅛ teaspoon sea salt
⅛ teaspoon turmeric powder
⅛ teaspoon freshly ground black pepper
2 tablespoons olive oil
2 tablespoons tahini
½ cup sauerkraut

Trim the middle stem of each collard leaf so it is not too thick. Place the collard leaves in a steamer and cook until softened, about 1 minute. Remove and set aside.

In a food processor, blend the zucchini, beans, avocado, onion, garlic, hemp seeds, parsley, vinegar, tamari, nutritional yeast, salt, turmeric, pepper, olive oil, and tahini until mostly smooth or to preferred consistency.

Lay a collard leaf on a clean surface. Scoop a portion of the hummus into the center of the wrap. Roll the collard like a burrito and slice in half. Continue until all the hummus is wrapped in collard leaves. Serve with a side of sauerkraut.

BUDDHA BOWLS

. . . .

(Vegan friendly without the eggs)

SERVES 2

2 cups cauliflower rice (see box on page 206)
2 tablespoons coconut oil, divided
1 cup halved Brussels sprouts or 2 cups shredded green
   cabbage
¼ teaspoon sea salt
½ cup shelled fresh organic edamame or canned black
   soybeans, drained
1½ tablespoons gluten-free tamari
½ tablespoon sesame oil
½ tablespoon chili sauce or sriracha
½ cup kimchi
2 scallions, roughly chopped
¼ cup hemp seeds
½ cup chopped cilantro
1 .17-ounce package seaweed snacks, torn into bite-sized
   pieces
2 radishes, sliced
2 hard-boiled eggs, halved (optional—leave out if vegan)
Extra-virgin olive oil (for drizzling)

If using store-bought cauliflower rice, place the rice in a large
skillet, add 2 tablespoons water, cover, and cook for 2 to 3
minutes on medium heat, or until slightly softened but not
mushy. Set aside. If you've prepared your own cauliflower
rice, this step is not necessary.

Heat 1 tablespoon coconut oil in the skillet over medium
heat. Sauté the Brussels sprouts (or cabbage) until softened but
not overcooked, about 3 minutes per side. Add the remaining
1 tablespoon oil and salt and cook, stirring, for another 3 minutes for the sprouts or just 1 more minute for the cabbage.

Lower heat and then stir in the beans, tamari, sesame oil, and chili sauce.

Remove from heat. Divide the cauliflower rice between 2 bowls. Arrange the cooked vegetables on top of each bowl. Divide the kimchi, scallions, hemp seeds, cilantro, seaweed, and radish between the bowls. Place an egg (if using) in the center of the bowl. Adjust salt and drizzle with oil.

DINNER RECIPES

ALMOND-CRUSTED CHICKEN TENDERS WITH CABBAGE LIME SLAW

SERVES 2

ALMOND-CRUSTED CHICKEN TENDERS

½ *cup almond flour*
½ *teaspoon sea salt*
½ *teaspoon freshly ground black pepper*
½ *teaspoon garlic powder*
½ *teaspoon onion powder*
½ *teaspoon dried rosemary*
¼ *teaspoon paprika*
½ *cup full-fat coconut milk*
8 *to 10 ounces boneless, skinless chicken tenders*

CABBAGE LIME SLAW

2 *cups shredded green cabbage*
1 *cup sprouts*
½ *medium white onion, sliced thin*
½ *cup chopped cilantro*
¼ *cup lime juice*
3 *tablespoons olive oil*
Sea salt
Freshly ground black pepper

Preheat oven to 400 degrees.

In a medium bowl, combine almond flour, salt, pepper, garlic powder, onion powder, rosemary, and paprika. Set aside.

Pour coconut milk into a shallow bowl. Dip chicken tenders in coconut milk. Dredge each tender in the almond flour mixture.

Arrange chicken on a parchment-lined baking sheet. Bake

for 7 minutes, flip the chicken, and continue cooking for another 7 to 8 minutes, or until chicken is golden on the outside and cooked through.

While chicken bakes, prepare the slaw. In a large bowl, combine cabbage, sprouts, onion, cilantro, lime juice, and oil. Season with salt and pepper.

Serve chicken with a large helping of slaw. It also tastes great with sides of ½ avocado, and a serving of pickled ginger.

GARDEN HARVEST BEEF STEW

SERVES 2

2 tablespoons olive oil
1 medium onion, diced
2 stalks celery, chopped
4 cloves garlic, minced
1 pound ground beef
2 sprigs oregano, leaves only, chopped
1 sprig of thyme, leaves only, chopped
1 teaspoon sea salt
1 teaspoon freshly ground black pepper
½ teaspoon cumin
½ teaspoon cayenne pepper
1 can (15 ounces) crushed tomatoes
5 cups beef or bone broth
1 cup broccoli florets
1 cup cauliflower florets
4 cups chopped kale
1 handful parsley, chopped

In a large soup or stock pot, heat olive oil over medium-high heat. Add onion, celery, and garlic. Cook for about 2 minutes or until onion and celery are slightly translucent.

Add beef and cook for another 7 to 8 minutes or until beef has mostly browned. Drain off any fat. Season with oregano, thyme, salt, pepper, cumin, and cayenne pepper. Stir in crushed tomatoes and broth.

Turn heat down to medium low and add broccoli, cauliflower, and kale. Cover and simmer for 15 minutes, or until broccoli and cauliflower are fork tender.

Serve hot, garnished with parsley and a side of ½ avocado and a half cup of sauerkraut, if desired.

CURRY SKILLET CHICKEN WITH COCONUT CILANTRO SAUCE AND CAULI-RICE

SERVES 2

CAULI-RICE

1½ tablespoons olive oil
4 cups cauliflower rice (see box on page 206)
Sea salt
Freshly ground black pepper

CHICKEN

1 teaspoon turmeric
½ teaspoon sea salt
½ teaspoon freshly ground black pepper
½ teaspoon cumin
½ teaspoon ground coriander
8 to 10 ounces boneless, skinless chicken thighs
1½ tablespoons ghee

SAUCE

½ cup coconut milk kefir
Juice and zest of 2 large limes
1 cup chopped cilantro
Sea salt
¼ cup chopped cashews

pickled ginger

Heat olive oil in a large skillet over medium-high heat. Add cauliflower rice. Season with salt and pepper. Cook for about 5 minutes on medium heat, stirring occasionally, until cauliflower is tender. Place in a medium bowl and set aside.

In a small bowl, combine turmeric, salt, pepper, cumin, and coriander. Evenly coat all sides of chicken with seasoning mixture. In the same skillet used for the rice, heat ghee over medium-high heat. Add the chicken to the skillet and cook for 4 to 5 minutes per side or until chicken is cooked through. Remove from heat.

In a blender or food processor, combine kefir, juice, zest, and cilantro. Blend until fully combined, and season lightly with salt.

Serve chicken on a bed of cauliflower rice with coconut sauce on top. Garnish with chopped cilantro and chopped cashews, and include a serving of pickled ginger on the side.

GINGER SALMON WITH CRISPY SKIN AND CRUCIFEROUS STIR-FRY

· ·

SERVES 2

STIR-FRY

2 tablespoons ghee
½ medium onion, sliced
2 cloves garlic, minced
1 cup broccoli florets
1 cup cauliflower florets
½ cup roughly chopped cabbage
Sea salt
Freshly ground black pepper

SALMON

2 filets (4 to 5 ounces each) wild-caught salmon with
  skin on
Sea salt
2 tablespoons coconut oil, melted
1 tablespoon grated fresh ginger
2 tablespoons coconut aminos
¼ cup sliced almonds, toasted

Heat ghee in a large wok or skillet over medium-high heat. Add onion and garlic and cook for about 2 minutes, or until onion is slightly translucent. Add broccoli, cauliflower, and cabbage. Season with salt and pepper and cook, stirring occasionally, for 5 to 6 minutes, or until veggies are fork tender. Set aside.

Pat both sides of salmon filets dry with a paper towel. Season both sides with salt. Put coconut oil in a cast-iron skillet or nonstick pan. Place salmon, skin side down, in the pan. Place it on the stove over medium-high heat. Cook for 3 to 4 minutes, gently pressing down on the salmon with a spatula to ensure that the skin is getting crispy. Cook for another 3 to 4 minutes or until fish is mostly opaque in color.

Carefully flip the salmon, then remove pan from heat. Leave salmon in hot pan to continue cooking for another 1 to 2 minutes.

In a small bowl, combine melted coconut oil, ginger, and coconut aminos. Whisk well; adjust seasoning.

Serve salmon with a big scoop of the stir-fried veggies, drizzle some of the ginger sauce over the top, and garnish with toasted almond slices. As side dishes, include ½ avocado and a serving of kimchi on each plate, if desired.

FISH TACOS WITH AVOCADO SALSA AND BROCCOLI SLAW

SERVES 2

SLAW

1½ cups broccoli slaw mix (can be found in most produce departments)
½ cup thinly shredded red cabbage
½ cup sprouts
¼ cup lime juice
2 tablespoons olive oil
Sea salt
Freshly ground black pepper

SALSA

1 avocado, pitted and cubed
1 mango, peeled, pitted, and cubed
½ small red onion, diced
2 medium vine-ripened tomatoes, chopped
½ cup chopped cilantro
Juice of 2 limes
Sea salt

TACOS

¾ teaspoon sea salt
½ teaspoon freshly ground black pepper
½ teaspoon garlic powder
½ teaspoon paprika
½ teaspoon cumin
¼ teaspoon chili powder
¼ teaspoon onion powder
¼ teaspoon cayenne pepper
10 ounces cod or other firm-fleshed white fish
1½ tablespoons ghee
4 to 6 whole cabbage leaves

In a large bowl, combine slaw mix, cabbage, sprouts, lime juice, and olive oil. Season with salt and pepper and toss. Cover and refrigerate.

In a medium bowl, combine avocado, mango, onion, tomatoes, cilantro, and lime juice. Toss and season lightly with salt.

In a small bowl, combine salt, pepper, garlic powder, paprika, cumin, chili powder, onion powder, and cayenne. Pat fish dry on all sides with a paper towel, and then season evenly on all sides with spice mixture.

Heat ghee in a medium cast-iron pan or nonstick skillet over medium-high heat. Add fish and cook for about 3 minutes per side, or until spices begin to turn dark brown and fish flakes easily with a fork.

Serve fish in a cabbage "taco" with slaw and salsa. Include a serving of pickled ginger on each plate if desired.

ONE-POT ROASTED CHICKEN
AND VEGGIES WITH CARAMELIZED LEMONS

SERVES 2

1 cup broccoli florets
1 cup cauliflower florets
1 cup chopped red cabbage
1 lemon, sliced thinly, with seeds removed
3 cloves garlic, sliced thinly
1 small onion, sliced
¼ cup olive oil, divided
2 sprigs thyme, leaves only
2 sprigs rosemary, leaves only
Sea salt
Freshly ground black pepper
10 ounces bone-in chicken thighs
Toasted almonds (optional)
Sauerkraut (optional)

Preheat oven to 350 degrees.

In a Dutch oven or braising pan, layer broccoli, cauliflower, cabbage, lemon, garlic, and onion. Drizzle with 3 tablespoons olive oil and toss gently. Add thyme and rosemary and season with salt and pepper.

Place chicken on top of veggies, skin side up. Drizzle with remaining olive oil and season with salt and pepper. Place in oven and roast for 20 minutes. Baste the chicken with the oil and juices in the pan. Cook for another 25 to 30 minutes or until chicken is cooked through and lemons have become caramelized.

Serve chicken with the veggies and lemon slices. Drizzle everything with the pan juices. Serve with toasted almonds and sauerkraut if desired.

Pro tip: Save bones from chicken to make bone broth.

GARLIC LIME MEATBALLS
WITH KIMCHI FRIED CAULI-RICE

SERVES 2

MEATBALLS

10 ounces ground beef
3 cloves garlic, minced
Juice and zest of 1 lime
⅓ cup almond flour
2 tablespoons olive oil
¼ cup finely chopped cilantro
½ small onion, finely diced
1 teaspoon sea salt
½ teaspoon freshly ground black pepper

KIMCHI FRIED CAULI-RICE

1 tablespoon olive oil
2 cloves garlic, minced
½ small onion, sliced
1 cup chopped kimchi
1 tablespoon grated fresh ginger
2 tablespoons coconut aminos
2 heads baby bok choy, leaves separated
3 cups cauliflower rice (see box on
  page 206)
Sea salt
Freshly ground black pepper
2 green onions, sliced

2 tablespoons toasted nuts

Preheat oven to 400 degrees.

In a large bowl, combine all ingredients for meatballs. Using your hands, make 2- to 3-inch meatballs and arrange them on a parchment-lined baking sheet.

Bake meatballs for 20 to 25 minutes, turning them about every 5 to 6 minutes.

While meatballs cook, prepare the fried rice. Heat oil in a large wok or skillet over medium-high heat. Add garlic and onion and cook for about 1 minute. Add kimchi and cook for another 2 minutes. Stir in ginger, coconut aminos, and bok choy and cook for about 2 minutes. Add cauliflower, season with salt and pepper, and cook for 3 to 4 minutes, or until cauliflower is tender. Garnish with green onions.

Serve fried cauliflower rice with meatballs and a serving of toasted nuts.

NOT YOUR MAMA'S CABBAGE SOUP

SERVES 2

5 to 6 cups bone broth
3 cloves garlic, minced
1 small jalapeño, seeded and minced
2 tablespoons grated fresh ginger
1 leek, white and pale green parts only, chopped
2 stalks celery, chopped
¼ cup lemon juice
2½ cups chopped cabbage
1 cup cauliflower florets
10 ounces skinless, boneless chicken breast, cubed
1½ teaspoons sea salt
1 teaspoon freshly ground black pepper
2 cups chopped bok choy
3 cups spinach, kale, or other dark leafy greens
½ cup chopped parsley
2 cups broccoli spiralized into "noodles" or sliced and
   boiled until tender

Combine broth, garlic, jalapeño, ginger, leek, celery, lemon juice, cabbage, cauliflower, chicken, salt, and pepper in a large slow cooker. Cover and cook on high for 2½ hours.

Add bok choy and spinach, cover, and cook for another 30 minutes. Stir in parsley and adjust seasoning.

Serve soup in a bowl over 1 cup prepared broccoli "noodles." On the side, include a serving of nuts and pickled ginger if desired.

CHINESE CASHEW CHICKEN LETTUCE WRAPS

SERVES 2

2 tablespoons coconut aminos
1 tablespoon cashew butter
⅓ cup low-sodium chicken broth
1½ tablespoons olive oil
3 cloves garlic, minced
½ onion, chopped
1 stalk celery, chopped
1 cup chopped broccoli
10 ounces ground chicken
1 tablespoon grated fresh ginger
1 teaspoon chili paste
2 cups spinach
⅓ cup chopped cashews
Sea salt
Freshly ground black pepper
4 to 6 butter lettuce leaves
1 handful cilantro, chopped
1 lime, cut into wedges
Pickled ginger (optional)

Combine coconut aminos, cashew butter, and broth in a small bowl. Whisk until fully blended. Set aside.

Heat olive oil in a large wok or skillet. Add garlic, onion, celery, and broccoli. Cook for 2 to 3 minutes. Add chicken, ginger, and chili paste. Cook, stirring, for about 5 minutes, or until chicken is nearly cooked through.

Add cashew butter mixture. Stir to combine, and add spinach and cashews. Season with salt and pepper. Cook for about 2 minutes, or until spinach has wilted.

Serve chicken mixture on lettuce leaves with cilantro on top and lime wedges on the side. Include some pickled ginger on each plate if desired.

LEMON POACHED FISH
WITH GARLICKY BEET GREENS

SERVES 2

FISH

1½ tablespoons ghee
1 small shallot, minced
1 clove garlic, minced
2 cups water
Juice and zest of 1 large lemon
½ teaspoon sea salt
½ teaspoon freshly ground black pepper
2 (5-ounce) halibut filets (or other firm-fleshed white fish)

BEET GREENS

1 tablespoon olive oil
1 bunch beet greens, chopped
2 cloves garlic, minced
½ teaspoon sea salt
½ teaspoon crushed red pepper flakes
⅓ cup sliced almonds

1 cup sauerkraut

Heat ghee in a large skillet over medium-high heat. Add shallot and garlic and cook for about 2 minutes. Reduce heat to medium and add water, lemon juice and zest, sea salt, and black pepper.

Reduce heat to low. Add fish, cover, and cook at a simmer for 10 minutes, or until fish is cooked through and flakes easily with a fork.

Remove fish from pan and continue to cook sauce in pan on medium-high heat for another 10 to 15 minutes, or until it thickens.

While you wait for sauce to reduce, cook the greens. Heat

olive oil in a large skillet over medium heat. Add beet greens, garlic, sea salt, and red pepper flakes. Cook until greens are tender, about 5 minutes. Stir in almonds and remove from heat.

Serve fish with beet greens, and drizzle reduction over fish. Include a half cup of sauerkraut on each plate.

GARLIC ROASTED CABBAGE AND CHICKEN

SERVES 2

3 tablespoons olive oil
Juice of 1 lemon
3 cloves garlic, minced
½ small head of cabbage, sliced into 2-inch rounds
½ red onion, sliced
10 ounces bone-in chicken thighs
1 sprig thyme, leaves only, chopped
1 sprig rosemary, leaves only, chopped
1 teaspoon sea salt
1 teaspoon freshly ground black pepper

Preheat oven to 375 degrees.

In a small bowl, whisk olive oil, lemon juice, and garlic.

On a greased, rimmed baking sheet, place cabbage rounds and scatter onion on top. Top with chicken thighs. Pour oil mixture over chicken and vegetables. Scatter thyme and rosemary evenly on top and season with salt and pepper.

Roast for 35 to 40 minutes, or until cabbage is tender and chicken is cooked through.

Serve with nuts and pickled ginger on the side, if desired.

TURMERIC MEATBALLS
WITH PARSLEY AND SPROUTS SLAW

. . . .

SERVES 2

MEATBALLS

1½ tablespoons olive oil

10 ounces ground beef

⅓ cup almond or coconut flour

3 cloves garlic, minced

½ cup finely chopped cilantro

1 tablespoon grated fresh ginger

1½ teaspoons ground turmeric

1 teaspoon sea salt

1 teaspoon cumin

½ teaspoon freshly ground black pepper

½ teaspoon coriander

¼ teaspoon cayenne pepper

¼ teaspoon cinnamon

SLAW

Juice of 1 large lemon

½ jalapeño, seeded and roughly chopped

⅓ cup full-fat coconut milk

½ teaspoon sea salt

1½ cups chopped parsley

1 cup sprouts

½ cup finely shredded red cabbage

1 small shallot, thinly sliced

Preheat oven to 400 degrees.

In a large bowl, combine all ingredients for meatballs. Using your hands, make 2-inch balls and arrange them on a parchment-lined baking sheet. Bake for about 20 minutes, rotating pan every 5 minutes.

While meatballs cook, prepare the slaw. In a blender, combine lemon juice, jalapeño, coconut milk, and salt. Blend until smooth.

In a large bowl, combine parsley, sprouts, cabbage, and shallots. Dress with coconut milk mixture and toss.

Serve meatballs with a big helping of slaw, and a side of avocado and pickled ginger, if desired.

COCONUT GINGER CHICKEN
WITH CILANTRO CAULI-RICE

SERVES 2

CHICKEN

2 tablespoons olive oil
3 cloves garlic, minced
2 tablespoons grated fresh ginger
½ onion, sliced
½ jalapeño, seeded and roughly chopped
1½ cups low-sodium chicken broth
Juice of 2 large limes
1 teaspoon sea salt
8 to 10 ounces skinless, boneless chicken breasts, cubed
1 cup broccoli florets
1 bell pepper (any color), seeded and sliced
½ cup full-fat coconut milk

CAULI-RICE

1½ tablespoons coconut oil
3 cups cauliflower rice (see box on page 206)
Sea salt
Freshly ground black pepper
Juice of 1 lime
½ cup chopped cilantro

Heat olive oil in a large skillet over medium-high heat. Add garlic, ginger, onion, and jalapeño. Cook for about 3 minutes or until fragrant, then deglaze the pan with the broth and lime juice.

Turn heat to low and add salt, chicken, broccoli, bell pepper, and coconut milk. Cover and simmer for 10 to 15 minutes, or until chicken is cooked through and veggies are fork-tender.

While chicken cooks, prepare cauli-rice. Heat coconut oil in a large skillet over medium-high heat, add cauliflower, and season with salt and pepper. Cook for about 5 minutes, or until cooked through. Stir in lime juice and cilantro and remove from heat.

Serve chicken and veggies, along with their sauce, over cilantro cauli-rice. Include a serving of toasted almonds and kimchi with each plate, if desired.

CABBAGE ROLL STEW

SERVES 2

8 ounces ground beef, browned
3 cloves garlic, minced
1 onion, chopped
1 stalk celery, chopped
2½ cups chopped cabbage
1 cup cauliflower rice (see box on page 206)
1 can (15 ounces) crushed tomatoes
4 cups beef or bone broth
1 tablespoon apple cider vinegar
1 tablespoon tomato paste
1 teaspoon sea salt
1 teaspoon freshly ground black pepper
½ teaspoon cumin
1 bay leaf

In a slow cooker, combine all ingredients. Cook on high for 3 to 4 hours. Remove bay leaf before serving.

Serve with sides of nuts and sauerkraut, if desired.

SPICED HALIBUT
WITH CRUNCHY CITRUS SALAD

. . . .

SERVES 2

HALIBUT

1 teaspoon sea salt

½ teaspoon freshly ground black pepper

½ teaspoon garlic powder

½ teaspoon onion powder

½ teaspoon cayenne pepper

¼ teaspoon chili powder

¼ teaspoon paprika

2 filets (5 ounces each) halibut or other firm-fleshed white fish

1 lime, cut into wedges

SALAD

1 head romaine lettuce, chopped

2 Persian cucumbers, sliced

1 small shallot, thinly sliced

2 radishes, thinly sliced

½ cup chopped cilantro

¼ cup MCT oil

Juice of 1 lemon

Juice of 1 lime

½ teaspoon sea salt

Preheat outdoor grill to medium-high heat.

In a small bowl, combine salt, pepper, garlic powder, onion powder, cayenne, chili powder, and paprika. Pat fish dry on all sides with a paper towel and evenly season with spice mixture.

Grease the grill grate and then place fish skin side down. Cook for about 5 minutes, then gently flip and cook for another 3 to 4 minutes. Remove from grill and set aside.

In a large bowl, combine lettuce, cucumbers, shallot, radishes, and cilantro and toss. In a small bowl, whisk together remaining ingredients (oil through salt). Dress salad with oil mixture.

Serve fish with a couple of wedges of lime, a generous helping of salad, and include a serving of avocado and pickled ginger, if desired.

SHEET PAN HERBY CHICKEN WITH CRUCIFEROUS VEGGIES

SERVES 2

2 cups halved Brussels sprouts
1 bunch radishes, halved
1 cup cauliflower florets
10 ounces boneless, skinless chicken thighs
3 tablespoons olive oil
Juice of 1 large lemon
1 sprig rosemary, leaves only, chopped
1 sprig thyme, leaves only, chopped
1 sprig oregano, leaves only, chopped
1 teaspoon sea salt
1 teaspoon freshly ground black pepper
1 teaspoon garlic powder
½ teaspoon onion powder
⅓ cup toasted sliced almonds

½ cup sauerkraut

Preheat oven to 375 degrees.

On a greased, rimmed sheet pan, arrange Brussels sprouts, radishes, cauliflower, and chicken. In a small bowl, combine oil and lemon juice. Evenly drizzle oil mixture over veggies and chicken. Season with rosemary, thyme, oregano, salt, pepper, garlic powder, and onion powder.

Bake 35 to 50 minutes, or until veggies are tender and chicken is cooked through. Garnish with almonds. Serve with a half cup of sauerkraut.

WHITE "KETO-NEY BEAN" STIR-FRY

(Vegan friendly)

SERVES 2

¼ *cup avocado oil*
2 *cloves garlic, minced*
2 *small zucchini, chopped*
2 *cups broccoli florets*
½ *teaspoon dried oregano*
½ *teaspoon crushed fennel seed*
¼ *teaspoon sea salt*
1 *cup canned white kidney beans, drained*
½ *avocado, sliced*
2 *tablespoons hemp seeds*
2 *teaspoons olive oil*
¼ *cup chopped parsley*
½ *cup sauerkraut*

Heat avocado oil over medium-high in a soup pot. Add garlic and cook, stirring, until fragrant, about 1 minute. Stir in zucchini, broccoli, oregano, fennel seed, and salt. Cook until vegetables soften, about 5 minutes.

Reduce heat to low, add beans, and cook for about 5 minutes, or until flavors come together.

Plate vegetable mixture and top with avocado and hemp seeds. Drizzle with oil and garnish with parsley. Adjust seasoning. Serve with sauerkraut on the side.

CASHEW CURRY WITH VEGETABLES OVER KETO "RICE"

(Vegan friendly)

SERVES 2

¼ cup raw cashews
1 teaspoon curry powder, divided
¼ teaspoon sea salt, divided
¾ cup Keto Alkaline Broth (page 221), divided
1 tablespoon coconut ghee
½ shallot, minced
2 cloves garlic, minced
1 cup spinach or bok choy
½ zucchini, diced
¼ red bell pepper, diced
½ cup canned black soybeans, drained, or 1 package
  (4 ounces) tempeh cut into ¼-inch thick cubes
1½ teaspoons apple cider vinegar
1 cup cauliflower rice (see box on page 206) or Wonder
  Noodles (shirataki noodles) cooked as directed
¼ cup roasted cashews

Make cashew cream: Soak cashews in 1 cup boiling water for 1 hour. Drain cashews and place in a blender. Add ½ teaspoon curry powder, ⅛ teaspoon salt, and 2 tablespoons broth and blend until smooth, periodically scraping down the sides of the blender with a small spatula. Add additional broth, 1 tablespoon at a time, to thin out cream as necessary. Measure out ½ cup cream. Store leftover cream in a glass jar in the refrigerator for up to 5 days.

Heat ghee in a skillet over medium heat. Add shallot and sauté 2 minutes; then add garlic, spinach, zucchini, bell pepper, and beans or tempeh. Cook, stirring frequently, until vegetables start to soften, about 5 minutes.

Lower heat. Stir in remaining broth, remaining curry powder, remaining salt, and vinegar and simmer for 5 minutes. Adjust the seasoning and remove from heat.

Place a serving of "rice" or noodles in each bowl. Top with curry and drizzle a generous amount of cashew cream over the top. Top with roasted cashews.

ZUCCHINI NOODLES
WITH WALNUT ROMESCO SAUCE

(Vegan friendly)

SERVES 2

1 jar (3½ ounces) roasted red peppers, drained
3 cherry tomatoes
1 cup Swiss chard leaves (no stems), steamed
½ cup walnuts
¼ cup parsley
½ cup fresh basil leaves
1 tablespoon olive oil
¼ teaspoon sea salt
¼ teaspoon freshly ground black pepper
1 clove garlic
1½ teaspoons apple cider vinegar
1 medium zucchini, spiralized

Combine red peppers, tomatoes, chard, walnuts, parsley, basil, olive oil, salt, pepper, garlic, and vinegar in a blender and blend until relatively smooth; small bits of walnut will remain.

Heat sauce in small saucepan over medium heat. Serve over zucchini noodles.

CAULIFLOWER "GNOCCHI" WITH PESTO AND WHITE BEANS

(Vegan friendly without the egg)

SERVES 2

GNOCCHI

>   3 cups cauliflower florets
>   ¼ cup coconut flour, plus extra for dusting
>   1 egg (vegan: 1 flax egg—mix 1 tablespoon ground flax
>   seeds with 3 tablespoons water and let stand 5 minutes)
>   ½ teaspoon sea salt, divided
>   2 tablespoons olive oil, divided

PESTO

>   ½ cup fresh basil leaves
>   ¼ cup fresh dandelion greens or parsley
>   1½ teaspoons nutritional yeast
>   ¼ cup hemp seeds
>   1 clove garlic
>   ⅛ teaspoon freshly ground black pepper

>   1 cup canned white kidney beans, drained
>   ½ cup sauerkraut

Preheat oven to 425 degrees.

Steam the cauliflower until fork-tender, about 3 to 5 minutes. Lay on a paper towel to drain and cool. Once the cauliflower is cool, twist and squeeze cauliflower to get out as much water as possible.

Transfer the cauliflower to a food processor and process until creamy. Add flour, egg, and ¼ teaspoon salt, and process again until it forms a dough. Add a little more flour if the dough is too loose.

Transfer the dough (it will be sticky) to a lightly floured cutting board and form a ball. Divide the ball into 4 equal parts. Roll each section with your hands to form a long rope about 1 inch in diameter. Slice the rope into ½-inch pieces. Repeat until all the dough is rolled and cut.

Line a baking sheet with parchment paper and grease the parchment. Place the gnocchi on the baking sheet in a single layer, drizzle with 1 tablespoon of oil, and bake 15 minutes. Flip gnocchi and bake 10 to 15 minutes more. Remove from oven and set aside.

While the gnocchi is roasting, make the pesto. Combine basil, dandelion greens or parsley, nutritional yeast, hemp seeds, garlic, salt, and pepper in a food processor and process 1 minute. With the processor running, drizzle in 1 tablespoon olive oil. Pulse 1 to 2 minutes more, until smooth.

Toss the gnocchi, pesto, and white kidney beans together and serve with a half cup of sauerkraut.

MASSAGED KALE SALAD
WITH ALMOND MISO DRESSING

. . . .

(Vegan friendly)

SERVES 2

SALAD

3 cups roughly chopped kale leaves (no stems)
¼ teaspoon sea salt, divided
½ cup non-GMO organic shelled edamame
2 tablespoons pumpkin seeds
½ cucumber, sliced thinly
¼ large carrot, shredded

DRESSING

1 tablespoon white miso paste
1 tablespoon unsweetened almond butter
¼ teaspoon monkfruit (optional)
1½ teaspoons raw apple cider vinegar or kefir
2 tablespoons olive oil
½ teaspoon grated fresh ginger

In a large bowl, combine kale and ⅛ teaspoon salt. With clean hands, massage the kale until it is wilted but not soggy. Add the edamame, pepitas, cucumber, and carrot. Set aside.

To make the dressing, whisk together miso, almond butter, monkfruit if using, vinegar or kefir, olive oil, ginger, and remaining salt until well combined. Dressing will be thick; if you prefer a thinner dressing, add filtered water, 1 tablespoon at a time.

Drizzle half of the dressing over the salad. Combine well and allow to sit for 10 minutes before serving. Divide salad between two plates and drizzle remaining dressing over each plate.

SNACKS AND SIDES

SPICY PUMPKIN SEED DIP

(Vegan friendly)

SERVES 2

1 cup raw hulled pumpkin seeds
1 medium vine-ripened tomato
½ jalapeño pepper, seeded
¼ cup chopped cilantro
¼ cup chopped parsley
2 cloves garlic
2 teaspoons apple cider vinegar
2 tablespoons olive oil
1 teaspoon sea salt

In a medium skillet over medium-high heat, toast pumpkin seeds, stirring constantly, for 2 to 4 minutes or until lightly golden. Remove from heat and allow to cool for several minutes.

In a food processor, combine pumpkin seeds and all remaining ingredients. Process until smooth.

Serve with a side of raw veggies for dipping (broccoli, cauliflower, etc.).

CUCUMBER AVOCADO
OPEN-FACED "SANDWICHES"

(Vegan friendly)

SERVES 2

1 avocado, sliced
1 small cucumber, halved and sliced lengthwise into
  ½ inch slices
Juice of 1 lime
1 teaspoon "everything" bagel seasoning

Arrange slices of avocado on top of each slab of cucumber. Drizzle with lime juice and sprinkle with seasoning.

LEMON DIJON DEVILED EGGS

SERVES 2

2 hard-boiled eggs, halved
2½ teaspoons paleo-approved mayonnaise
1 teaspoon Dijon mustard
½ teaspoon MCT oil
1 teaspoon lemon juice
½ teaspoon sea salt
¼ teaspoon paprika
1 teaspoon minced chives

Scoop yolks out of each half of egg and place into a medium bowl. Add mayonnaise, mustard, oil, lemon juice, salt, and paprika. Whisk until smooth.

Transfer mixture into a small plastic bag, cut a small hole in one corner, and squeeze the mixture into the center of each egg half. Garnish with chives.

QUICK FRIDGE PICKLES

(Vegan friendly)

SERVES 2

½ cup sliced cucumber
½ cup sliced radishes
¼ cup julienned carrots
½ medium red onion, thinly sliced
1 clove garlic, thinly sliced
½ teaspoon black peppercorns
½ teaspoon sea salt
1 cup apple cider vinegar
½ cup water

In a medium bowl, combine cucumber, radishes, carrot, onion, and garlic. Transfer to a jar and add peppercorns.

In the same bowl used for the veggies, combine salt, vinegar, and water. Whisk until salt is completely dissolved. Pour over veggies (make sure vegetables are packed down so liquid can cover them), seal, and place in refrigerator for at least 2 hours before serving.

Serve with avocado slices on the side.

KETO-GREEN N' OATMEAL

MAKES 2 SERVINGS

4 tablespoons coconut oil or ghee
1 cup liquid egg whites
2 cups unsweetened almond or coconut milk
½ cup full-fat coconut milk
2 cups cauliflower rice (see box on page 206)
2 tablespoons chia seeds
2 tablespoons hemp seeds
1 teaspoon pumpkin pie spice or cinnamon
1 teaspoon monkfruit or 1 teaspoon granulated stevia
1 scoop Dr. Anna Cabeca Keto-Green Meal Replacement
  or similar product

Warm the oil in a small saucepan over medium heat. Add the egg whites and cook, stirring, until scrambled.

Add the milk, cauliflower, chia, hemp, pumpkin pie spice, and sweetener and stir.

Remove from heat and stir in protein powder. Add water, 1 tablespoon at a time, if you prefer a thinner consistency.

DESSERTS

MANGO COCONUT SORBET

(Vegan friendly)

SERVES 2

1 cup frozen mango
1 cup full-fat coconut milk
½ teaspoon pure vanilla extract
¼ cup unsweetened coconut flakes, toasted

Combine mango, coconut milk, and vanilla in a blender and blend until smooth. Pour contents into a freezer-safe container, seal, and place in the freezer for at least 2 hours before serving. Scoop into dishes and garnish with coconut flakes.

CARDAMOM CASHEW FAT BOMBS

(Vegan friendly)

SERVES 2

½ cup raw cashews
¼ cup almond flour
3 tablespoons coconut butter, divided
1 tablespoon coconut oil
1 teaspoon pure vanilla extract
1 teaspoon lemon zest
½ teaspoon cardamom
½ teaspoon ground ginger
2 dates, pitted

In a food processor, pulse cashews until ground. Add almond flour, 1½ tablespoons coconut butter, coconut oil, vanilla, lemon zest, cardamom, ginger, and dates. Blend until thoroughly combined. Roll cashew mixture into 2- to 3-inch balls and set aside.

In a microwave or in a small pot on the stove, gently heat remaining coconut butter just until it's a liquid consistency; be careful not to burn it.

Drizzle coconut butter over the cashew balls. Let rest for 15 minutes or until coconut butter cools to room temperature.

PINEAPPLE LIME GRANITA

(Vegan friendly)

SERVES 2

1 cup pineapple chunks
¼ cup lime juice
Zest of 1 lime

Combine all ingredients in a blender and blend until smooth. Transfer mixture to a freezer-safe shallow pan. Place in freezer for 35 to 40 minutes, then remove and scrape with a fork to create frozen pea-sized pieces. Repeat this 2 or 3 times.

After the last scrape, place back in freezer and allow to sit untouched for at least 2 hours before serving.

DARK CHOCOLATE CHIA PUDDING

(Vegan friendly)

SERVES 2

½ cup unsweetened almond or coconut milk
2 tablespoons chia seeds
2 tablespoons hemp seeds
1 tablespoon cacao powder
1½ teaspoons monkfruit
½ cup coconut cream
1 tablespoon MCT oil
1 scoop Dr. Anna Cabeca Keto-Green Meal Replacement
*   or similar product*
¼ cup chopped papaya, mango, or pineapple, or fresh
*   berries*

Place milk in a glass container. Stir in chia and hemp seeds and then the cacao powder, monkfruit sweetener, cream, and oil. Refrigerate at least 2 hours and preferably overnight.

Before serving, stir in the protein powder. Serve cold, topped with fruit.

APPENDIX B

Keto-Green 16 Resources

dranna.com/KetoGreenBook

Keto pH Test Strips: dranna.com; Simplex Health,
    simplexhealth.co.uk
Hydrion pH Paper: amazon.co.uk
KETO-MOJO Blood Ketone and Glucose Testing
    Meter Kit or Precision X-tra blood ketone monitor:
    amazon.co.uk
FreeStyle Libre 14-day system for continuing blood sugar
    monitoring: contact freestylelibre.co.uk

Argentyn Silver, amazon.co.uk
Dr. Anna Cabeca's Better Brain & Sleep (magnesium L-
    threonate)
Dr. Anna Cabeca's Keto-Alkaline Detox Support
Dr. Anna Cabeca's Keto-Alkaline Protein Shake (0g sugar)
Dr. Anna Cabeca Keto-Green Meal Replacement (0g sugar)
Dr. Anna Cabeca Mighty Maca Plus
Dr. Anna Cabeca's Vida Optimal Balance (hormone-
    balancing herbal formula)
Opti-Lean Fiber from xymogen.com
Probiotics: Probio ENT, chewable probiotic by Xymogen;
    Probio Max BeLive probiotic gummies
Spore-containing probiotics: just Thrive probiotic or
    Megasporebiotic by Microbiome Labs
Vital-Zymes chewable digestive enzymes by Klaire labs,
    amazon.co.uk

HIGH-QUALITY MULTIVITAMINS AND NUTRACEUTICAL COMPANIES

designsforhealth.com

proactivehealthcare.co.uk

pharmaquipe.co.uk

NATURAL SOLUTIONS FOR WOMEN BY DR. ANNA

Dr. Anna Cabeca's Julva feminine cream

Dr. Anna Cabeca's PuraBalance PPR cream

KITCHENWARE AND COOKING TOOLS

Bamboo cutting boards

Cast-iron skillets

Ceramic skillets

CorningWare

Glass jars and storage bowls

Glass ovenware, like Pyrex

Hamilton Beach Set & Forget Slow Cooker (It is free of lead, which many slow cookers contain.)

NutriBullet and Veggie Bullet (love these!)

Radiant Life 14-Stage Biocompatible Water Purification System

Wusthof Knives

Vitamix

NONTOXIC HOUSEHOLD PRODUCTS

EC3 laundry detergent, mold cleaner, and cleaning products

Seventh Generation

Thieves Oil cleaning products

White vinegar

WATER FILTERS

Berkey Water Filter (when installing under the sink is not
  possible)
Finer Filters, finer.filters.co.uk
For lead removal, you want to be looking for NSF/ANSI
  Standard 53 for pitcher, faucet, countertop, refrigerator,
  or in-line filters
Vollara.com (living water sink system and laundry system)

HELPFUL WEBSITES

dranna.com (see dranna.com/resources)
drmasley.com (Steven Masley, MD)
drperlmutter.com (David Perlmutter, MD, the empowering
  neurologist)
drritamarie.com (nutritional endocrinology by Ritamarie
  Loscalzo, DC)
EWG.org (Environmental Working Group)
functionalmedicine.org (Finding a Functional Medicine Doc)
IFM.org (Institute of Functional Medicine and Finding a
  Functional Medicine Doctor)
quicksilverscientific.com
PCCARX.com (For compounding pharmacies)
jjvirgin.com
drkellyann.com

CLINICAL LABORATORIES (THE ONES I RELY ON FOR TESTING)

(Array 4) and Permeability (Array 2)
Cell Science Systems GmbH: Alcat Food Sensitivity Test
Cyrex Labs: Gluten-Associated Cross-Reactive Foods and
  Food Sensitivity
Detoxification
Genova Diagnostics Europe: Nutrition testing, Hormones,
  Estrogen, Detoxification

Invivo Clinical; Gi-MAP (stool test)

Pathways

Precision Analytics: Urinary Testing for Hormones and Nutrition and Estrogen

Quicksilver Scientific: quicksilverscientific.com for Heavy Metals Testing

Smart Nutrition: Adrenal Stress Index

23andMe: Ancestry and Health

Ubiome.com: Jane test (a vaginal health test)

UltaLabTests.com/dranna (for my recommended blood panels)

FOOD SITES I RECOMMEND

Fieldandflower.co.uk (for wild-caught seafood and grass-fed beef)

Raw-Wild.co.uk

Wholefoodsmarket.co.uk

OTHER ITEMS I'VE FOUND HELPFUL

Heartmath.com

Muse.com

Xalm weighted blanket

Sunlighten infrared sauna

Wholetones.com

APPENDIX C

References

CHAPTER 1: SO . . . YOU CAN'T LOSE WEIGHT?

Villareal, D. T., and J. O. Holloszy. 2004. Effect of DHEA on abdominal fat and insulin action in elderly women and men: a randomized controlled trial. *JAMA* 292: 2243–2248.

CHAPTER 2: JUST GIVE ME 16 DAYS

Ahuja, K. D., et al. 2003. Effects of two lipid-lowering, carotenoid-controlled diets on the oxidative modification of low-density lipoproteins in free-living humans. *Clinical Science* 105: 355–361.

Bes-Rastrollo, M., et al. 2009. Prospective study of nut consumption, long-term weight change, and obesity risk in women. *American Journal of Clinical Nutrition* 89: 1913–1919.

Bozzetto, L., et al. 2016. Extra-virgin olive oil reduces glycemic response to a high–glycemic index meal in patients with type 1 diabetes: a randomized controlled trial. *Diabetes Care* 39: 518–524.

Caciano, S., et al. 2015. Effects of dietary acid load on exercise metabolism and anaerobic exercise performance. *Journal of Sports Science & Medicine* 14: 364–371.

Della, L. G., et al. 2016. Diet-induced acidosis and alkali supplementation. *International Journal of Food Sciences and Nutrition* 67: 754–761.

Ebbeling, C. B., et al. 2018. Effects of a low carbohydrate diet on energy expenditure during weight loss maintenance: randomized trial. *British Medical Journal* 363 (Nov 14): k4583.

Faure, A. M., et al. 2017. Gender-specific association between dietary acid load and total lean body mass and its dependency on protein intake in seniors. *Osteoporosis International* 28: 3451–3462.

Galvão, C. F., et al. 2014. Consumption of extra-virgin olive oil improves body composition and blood pressure in women with excess body fat: a randomized, double-blinded, placebo-controlled clinical trial. *European Journal of Clinical Nutrition* 57: 2445–2455.

Gomes, A. C., et al. 2017. The additional effects of a probiotic mix on abdominal adiposity and antioxidant status: a double-blind, randomized trial. *Obesity* 25: 30–38.

Kabiri, A., et al. 2016. Impact of olive oil–rich diet on serum omentin and adiponectin levels: a randomized cross-over clinical trial among overweight women. *International Journal of Food Sciences and Nutrition* 68: 560–568.

Kábrt, L., et al. 1990. Low-energy protein diet and starvation diet in the obese—effect on energy metabolism. *Czechoslovak Medicine* 13: 175–183.

Kim, E. K., et al. 2011. Fermented kimchi reduces body weight and improves metabolic parameters in overweight and obese patients. *Nutrition Research* 31: 436–443.

Lee, M., et al. 2016. Anthocyanin rich-black soybean testa improved visceral fat and plasma lipid profiles in overweight/obese Korean adults: a randomized controlled trial. *Journal of Medicinal Food* 19: 995–1003.

——, et al. 2017. Dietary anthocyanins against obesity and inflammation. *Nutrients* 9: E1089.

Moreno, B., et al. 2016. Obesity treatment by very low-calorie-ketogenic diet at two years: reduction in visceral fat and on the burden of disease. *Endocrine* 54: 681–690.

Ruggles, K. V., et al. 2018. Changes in the gut microbiota of urban subjects during an immersion in the traditional diet and lifestyle of a rainforest village. *mSphere* 29: 4.

Saslow, L. R., et al. 2017. Twelve-month outcomes of a randomized trial of a moderate-carbohydrate versus very low-carbohydrate diet in overweight adults with type 2 diabetes mellitus or prediabetes. *Nutrition & Diabetes* 7: 304.

Wigglesworth, V. B. 1924. Studies on ketosis: I. The relation between alkalosis and ketosis. *Biochemical Journal* 18: 1203–1216.

Williams, R. S., et al. 2016. The role of dietary acid load and mild metabolic acidosis in insulin resistance in humans. *Biochimie* 124: 171–177.

CHAPTER 3: THE 16 KETO-GREEN FOODS

Dreher, M. L., and A. J. Davenport. 2013. Hass avocado composition and potential health effects. *Critical Reviews in Food Science and Nutrition* 53: 738–750.

Haddad, E., et al. 2018. Postprandial gut hormone responses to Hass avocado meals and their association with visual analog scores in overweight adults: a randomized 3 × 3 crossover trial. *Eating Behaviors* 31: 35–40.

Han, J. R., et al. 2007. Effects of dietary medium-chain triglyceride on weight loss and insulin sensitivity in a group of moderately overweight free-living type 2 diabetic Chinese subjects. *Metabolism* 56: 985–991.

Kim, M., et al. 2015. Fish oil intake induces UCP1 upregulation in brown and white adipose tissue via the sympathetic nervous system. *Scientific Reports* 17: 18013.

Kinsella, R., et al. 2017. Coconut oil has less satiating properties than medium-chain triglyceride oil. *Physiology & Behavior* 179: 422–426.

Yoon-Mi, L., et al. 2017. Dietary anthocyanins against obesity and inflammation. *Nutrients* 9: 1089.

CHAPTER 4: THE FAT-LOSS POWER OF INTERMITTENT FASTING

Arnason, T. G., et al. Effects of intermittent fasting on health markers in those with type 2 diabetes: a pilot study. *World Journal of Diabetes* 8: 154–164.

Barnosky, A. R., et al. 2014. Intermittent fasting vs. daily calorie restriction for type 2 diabetes prevention: a review of human findings. *Translational Research* 164: 302–311.

Catenacci, V. A., et al. 2016. A randomized pilot study comparing zero-calorie alternate-day fasting to daily caloric restriction in adults with obesity. *Obesity* 24: 1874–1883.

Faris, M. A. E., et al. 2019. Effect of Ramadan diurnal fasting on visceral adiposity and serum adipokines in overweight and obese individuals. *Diabetes Research and Clinical Practice* 153: 166–175.

Marinac, C. R., et al. 2016. Prolonged nightly fasting and breast cancer prognosis. *JAMA Oncology* 2: 1049–1055.

Mattson, M. P., V. D. Longo, and M. Harvie. 2017. Impact of intermittent fasting on health and disease processes. *Ageing Research Reviews* 39: 46–58.

Mehrdad, A., et al. 2010. Short-term fasting induces profound neuronal autophagy. *Autophagy* 6: 702–710.

Nair, P. M., and P. G. Khawale. 2016. Role of therapeutic fasting in women's health: an overview. *Journal of Midlife Health* 7: 61–64.

Rothschild, J., et al. 2014. Time-restricted feeding and risk of metabolic disease: a review of human and animal studies. *Nutrition Reviews* 72: 308–318.

Varady, K. A. 2011. Intermittent versus daily calorie restriction: which diet regimen is more effective for weight loss? *Obesity Reviews* 12: e593–e601.

Webber, J., and I. A. MacDonald. 1994. The cardiovascular, metabolic and hormonal changes accompanying acute starvation in men and women. *British Journal of Nutrition* 71: 437–447.

Zarrinpar, A., et al. 2014. Diet and feeding pattern affect the diurnal dynamics of the gut microbiome. *Cell Metabolism* 20: 1006–1007.

Zubryzycki, A., et al. 2018. The role of intermittent fasting in treating obesity and type 2 diabetes. *Journal of Physiology and Pharmacology* 69: 663–683.

CHAPTER 5: THE BREAKTHROUGH KETO-GREEN 16 DIET PLAN

Mousa, H. A. 2016. Health effects of alkaline diet and water, reduction of digestive-tract bacterial load, and earthing. *Alternative Therapies in Health and Medicine* suppl. 1: 24–33.

CHAPTER 7: WEIGHT-CONTROL SUPPLEMENTS
THAT REALLY WORK

Aoe, S., et al. 2017. Effects of high β-glucan barley on visceral fat obesity in Japanese individuals: a randomized, double-blind study. *Nutrition* 42: 1–6.

Camfield, D. A., et al. 2013. The effects of multivitamin supplementation on diurnal cortisol secretion and perceived stress. *Nutrients* 5: 4429–4450.

Editor. 2003. Vitamin C: stress buster. *Psychology Today,* April 25.

Kamal, P. 2018. Maca; summary of maca. Examine.com, June 14, 2018. https://examine.com/supplements/maca.

Pooyandjoo, M., et al. 2016. The effect of (L-)carnitine on weight loss in adults: a systematic review and meta-analysis of randomized controlled trials. *Obesity Reviews* 17: 970–976.

Sanchez, M., et al. 2014. Effect of *Lactobacillus rhamnosus* CGMCC1.3724 supplementation on weight loss and maintenance in obese men and women. *British Journal of Nutrition* 111: 1507–1519.

Suarez, F., et al. 1999. Pancreatic supplements reduce symptomatic response of healthy subjects to a high fat meal. *Digestive Diseases and Sciences* 44: 1317–1321.

Szewczyk-Golec, K., et al. 2017. Melatonin supplementation lowers oxidative stress and regulates adipokines in obese patients on a calorie-restricted diet. *Oxidative Medicine and Cellular Longevity*, September 21 epub.

Ward, E. 2014. Addressing nutritional gaps with multivitamin and mineral supplements. *Nutrition Journal* 13: 72.

Willoughby, D., et al. 2018. Body composition changes in weight loss: strategies and supplementation for maintaining lean body mass, a brief review. *Nutrients* 10: 1876.

Zhang, Y. Y., et al. 2017. Efficacy of omega-3 polyunsaturated fatty acids supplementation in managing overweight and obesity: a meta-analysis of randomized clinical trials. *Journal of Nutrition, Health & Aging* 21: 187–192.

CHAPTER 8: NOT FOR WOMEN ONLY: GET YOUR MAN ON THIS PLAN!

Beauchet, O. 2006. Testosterone and cognitive function: current clinical evidence of a relationship. *European Journal of Endocrinology* 155: 773–781.

Carruba, G. 2007. Estrogen and prostate cancer: an eclipsed truth in an androgen-dominated scenario. *Journal of Cellular Biochemistry* 102: 899–911.

Cohen, P. G. 1999. The hypogonadal-obesity cycle: role of aromatase in modulating the testosterone-estradiol shunt—a major factor in the genesis of morbid obesity. *Medical Hypotheses* 52: 49–51.

Guneet, K. J., et al. 2013. Circulating estrone levels are associated prospectively with diabetes risk in men of the Framingham Heart Study. *Diabetes Care* 36: 2591–2596.

Masley, S. n.d. Does testosterone decrease or increase heart disease in men? DrMasley.com. https://drmasley.com/does-testosterone-decrease-or-increase-heart-disease-in-men.

Moffat, S. D. 2005. Effects of testosterone on cognitive and brain aging in elderly men. *Annals of the New York Academy of Sciences* 1055: 80–92.

Park, B. Y., et al. 2016. Is Internet pornography causing sexual dysfunctions? A review with clinical reports. *Behavioral Sciences* 6: 17.

Rebuffé-Scrive, M., et al. 1991. Effect of testosterone on abdominal adipose tissue in men. *International Journal of Obesity* 15: 791–795.

Urology Care Foundation. n.d. What is low testosterone? https://www.urologyhealth.org/urologic-conditions/low-testosterone.

CHAPTER 9: THE 16-MINUTE FITNESS PLAN

Colado, J. C., et al. 2009. Effects of aquatic resistance training on health and fitness in postmenopausal women. *European Journal of Applied Physiology* 106: 113–122.

Lu, Y. H., et al. 2016. Twelve-minute daily yoga regimen reverses osteoporotic bone loss. *Topics in Geriatric Rehabilitation* 32: 81–87.

Pascoe, M. C., et al. 2017. Yoga, mindfulness-based stress reduction and stress-related physiological measures: a meta-analysis. *Psychoneuroendocrinology* 86: 152–168.

Ring-Dimitriou, S., et al. 2008. Exercise modality and physical fitness in perimenopausal women. *European Journal of Applied Physiology* 105: 739–747.

Schaun, G. Z., et al. 2017. Acute effects of high-intensity interval training and moderate-intensity continuous training sessions on cardiorespiratory parameters in healthy young men. *European Journal of Applied Physiology* 117: 1437–1444.

Serrano, Guzmán, M., and M. E. Aguilar-Ferrándiz. 2016. Effectiveness of a flamenco and sevillanas program to enhance mobility, balance, physical activity, blood pressure, body mass, and quality of life in postmenopausal women living in the community in Spain: a randomized clinical trial. *Menopause* 23: 965–973.

SWAN Collaborators. n.d. Study of women's health across the nation, www.swanstudy.org.

Trapp, E. G., et al. 2008. The effects of high-intensity intermittent exercise training on fat loss and fasting insulin levels of young women. *International Journal of Obesity* 32: 684–691.

Wang, Y., et al. 2017. Tai chi exercise for the quality of life in a perimenopausal women organization: a systematic review. *Worldviews on Evidence-Based Nursing* 14: 294–305.

Zhang, J., et al. 2014. Effects of physical exercise on health-related quality of life and blood lipids in perimenopausal women: a randomized placebo-controlled trial. *Menopause* 21: 1269–1276.

CHAPTER 10: THE CLEAN 16

Kim, H. 2007. Effect of aromatherapy massage on abdominal fat and body image in post-menopausal women. *Taehan Kanho Hakhoe Chi* 37: 603–612.

Marcelle, M. R., et al. 2019. Growing resilience through interaction with nature: can group walks in nature buffer the effects of stressful life events on mental health? *International Journal of Environment Research and Public Health* 16: E986.

CHAPTER 11: DAY 17 AND BEYOND

An, R., and J. McCaffrey. 2016. Plain water consumption in relation to energy intake and diet quality among US adults, 2005–2012. *Journal of Human Nutrition and Dietetics* 29: 624–632.

Van Walleghen, E. L., et al. 2007. Pre-meal water consumption reduces meal energy intake in older but not younger subjects. *Obesity* 15: 93–99.

ACKNOWLEDGMENTS

When I published my first book, *The Hormone Fix,* I was thrilled by its reception and the fact that it became a *USA Today* bestseller. I was also thrilled that, right away, my publisher wanted this second book. I'm so glad for that encouragement. I honestly didn't think I could get it done in the requested short time frame, but with the help of supportive family, friends, and acquaintances, and after immense focus and love, here it is! I am grateful to so many.

I first want to acknowledge, with great love, my children, Brittany, Amanda, Amira, Garrett—in heaven—and Avamarie, all who have been by my side along the way. They have seen me, a single-mom entrepreneur, whittle away late nights and early mornings and yet be present for them. I am thrilled to see how they now support one another in such helpful, loving ways. This has given me the strength and ability to share my passions with you and the world.

I am indebted to all my clients who have followed my advice and encouragement and have been embracing the Keto-Green lifestyle and supporting one another. You all inspire me.

Maggie Greenwood, I am so grateful for your collaboration and writing skills—I absolutely love you and love working with you. I could not have done this without you.

To my literary agent, Heather Jackson, thank you for your encouragement and tenacity and gracious guidance and support in so many areas. This has been a fun journey with you.

I am deeply grateful to all those at Penguin Random House's Ballantine Books, especially Marnie Cochran, for skillfully overseeing this masterpiece. Thank you for your exceptional expertise and guidance.

To all my team at Dr. Anna Cabeca, I am so grateful to each and every one of you: Jamellette Diffott-Casiano, Lori Thomas, Connie Calhoun, Alexis Odum, Rosanna Alvarado, Jamy Casiano, Yael Goodman, Josh Koerpel, Courtney Webster, Shibani Subramanya, Andrew Way, Diane Blum, Chris Loch, Andreas Fried, David Stack, Amanda Hartwick, Rachel McGhie, Travis Ziegler, Adam Pixler, Randy Thebeau, Helen Dooley, and, of course, my daughters Brittany, Amira, and Amanda Claire Bivens.

To all of you, as my team, I am completely blessed by each and every one of you, your individual expertise, skill, and collaboration is exceptional. Thank you so much for all you do!

To our workout trainer, Vinay Khurana, thank you for keeping us fit locally. And to Caroline Ely: I am so grateful for your recipe support, as well as for these gorgeous pictures. You are so gifted.

To Chris Moncus, thanks for making my recipe videos and helping these beautiful recipes come to life.

To all my taste testers—Amanda, Brittany, Amira, Avamarie (especially with the desserts), Izzy, and Marigona—you have been a great help! Each and every one of you has become a great chef too.

Seeing the next generation of health-conscious individuals blossoming makes my heart sing.

To my PR team, the Butin Group—Mary, Kelly, Jade, Mary Eva, Madison: I am so grateful to each of you and all you do to bring this message out into the world and represent me.

Pamela Bruner, I am so grateful for your wisdom and support. Thank you also to my dear friends and colleagues who have encouraged me, helped me, and supported me along the way: Dr. David Perlmutter, JJ Virgin, Magdalena Wszelaki, Dr. Ellie Campbell, Dr. Angeli Akey, Hamida Lau, Aubrie Reedy, Mary Butin, Debbie Temmer, Yael Vilenski, Helene Burke, Dr. Lori Trefts, and all my Unicorns and Mindshare friends! I'm blessed to be part of these fabulous groups. And heartfelt thanks to Dr. Debra Shepherd, who like an angel came and took over my practice for a year after my son passed away and who enabled this journey that has now blessed hundreds of thousands of lives around the world. Bless you, all of you.

And to all you out there who are showing up for yourselves and for your families and all those you love, knowing that your magnificence is your blessing to yourself and others.

With much love and gratitude,

Dr. Anna

INDEX

mood swings, 10, 12, 54, 136
morning routine, 80
  meal plan, 89–94
  Vegan Keto-Green 16 diet, 100,
    105, 106–11
MPS (muscle protein synthesis),
  157
mTOR, 68
multivitamins, 117–19, 144
muscle mass, 14, 20, 33, 35, 36,
  67–68, 136, 148
Muscle Maven Smoothie, 212
muscle strength, 12, 14, 19, 21, 22
mushrooms, 112
mustard greens, 30

N.O. Max ER, 146
naps, 104
National Institutes of Health, 13
nature, 173–75
nausea, 28, 43
Neo40, 146
Neogenesis, 146
nervous systems, 5–6
nettles, 113
neurodegenerative diseases, 68
neuroendocrine vulnerability, xv,
  8–10
Neurology study, 51
neurotransmitters, 11, 137
New Naked, The (Fisch), 137–38
night sweats, 11, 12, 15, 136
nitric oxide, 146
non-genetically-modified (non-
  GMO) foods, 85
non-heme iron, 112
North Florida Integrative
  Medicine, Gainesville,
  Florida, xvi
Not Your Mama's Cabbage Soup,
  261
Nurses' Health Study, 55
nut milks, 61

Nutrition Journal, 117
Nutrition Research, 57
Nutrition study, 128
nuts, 16, 30, 47, 55–56, 96, 97,
  113, 193

Oatmeal, Keto-Green N', 285
obesity, x, 3, 17, 21, 44, 68, 86,
  119, 125, 133, 136
Obesity journal, 57, 66, 194
Obesity Reviews, 129
obesogens, 198–99
olive oil, 30, 47, 54–55, 61, 85, 96,
  193
olives, 17, 30
omega-3 fatty acids, 48, 49, 50,
  113, 130
omega-6 and omega-9 fatty
  acids, 49
One-Pot Roasted Chicken and
  Veggies with Caramelized
  Lemons, 258
onions, 52, 53, 97, 99
organic foods, 36, 50
orgasms, 19, 86, 137, 200
osteopenia, 136, 167
osteoporosis, 14, 88, 136, 166,
  167
Osteoporosis International
  study, 36
ovaries, 5, 134
overhead presses, 164
ox bile, 147
*Oxidative Medicine and Cellular
  Longevity,* 125
oxidative stress, 8
oxygen, xviii, 166
oxytocin, 5, 6, 14, 86, 119, 177,
  181, 182, 198, 200
  described, 19
  exercise and, 156
  signs of low, 19–20
oysters, 49, 144

ABOUT THE AUTHOR

ANNA CABECA, DO, OBGYN, FACOG, is an internationally acclaimed menopause and sexual health expert, global speaker, and pioneering promoter of women's health. She is Emory University–trained and triple board-certified in gynecology and obstetrics, integrative medicine, and antiaging and regenerative medicine. She is the author of *The Hormone Fix,* a diet and holistic lifestyle program for menopausal women.

Dr. Cabeca's areas of specialty include bioidentical hormone treatments and natural hormone-balancing strategies, and she has received extensive acclaim for her virtual transformational programs, including Women's Restorative Health, Sexual CPR, and Magic Menopause. She created the successful and popular alkaline superfoods drink Mighty Maca Plus and a top-selling, rejuvenating vulvar cream for women, Julva.

Dr. Cabeca was named 2018 Innovator of the Year by Mindshare, the number one conference for health and wellness influencers, and was also honored with the prestigious 2017 Alan P. Mintz Award, presented annually by the Age Management Medicine Group to an outstanding physician who displays clinical excellence and entrepreneurship.

Dr. Cabeca has reached hundreds of thousands of women around the globe, inspiring them to reclaim their optimal health and realize they can journey through menopause and find more purpose and pleasure than they ever dreamed possible. She has been interviewed by all major television networks and has been featured in *InStyle, HuffPost, First,* and *MindBodyGreen.* She balances her passion for women's health with faith, grace, and skill while raising four daughters on St. Simons Island, Georgia, and leading the nonprofit foundation she created in honor of her son, Garrett V. Bivens, who tragically died as a toddler.

Follow her journey on her blog at dranna.com.